M000201951

Clostridium difficile: A Patient's Guide

CLOSTRIDIUM DIFFICILE: A PATIENT'S GUIDE

CHRISTOPHER O'NEAL, PH.D. AND RAF RIZK, M.D.

ILLUSTRATIONS BY MARIANNE KHALIL

All rights reserved. Printed in the United States of America. No part of this publication may be reproduced or transmitted in any form or by any means, electronic or mechanical, including photocopy, recording, or any information storage and retrieval system, without permission in writing from the publisher.

Copyright © 2011 by Inner Workings Press

Published in 2011 in the United States of America by Inner Workings Press, 2335 Paseo Circulo, Tustin, CA 92782.

Find us on the World Wide Web at www.c-difficile-book.com

A CIP catalog record for this book is available from the Library of Congress.

ISBN 978-0-578-08913-3

Table of Contents

Acknowledgements

The authors and illustrator of this book would like to thank the friends and family who've stood by them whether they were sick or well. This book, a collaboration between a doctor and his patient, is a testament to the power these two parties have when they work together. It's dedicated to doctors and patients everywhere.

Chris would like to give special thanks to his wife and partner, Victoria, who suffered through C. diff with him, and beat C. diff with him. He also owes a debt a gratitude to his doctor and co-author, Dr. Raf Rizk, who stayed true to his patient over a very long haul. Thanks to the five patients who contributed their success stories to the book. Additionally, he is very grateful to Beverly and Johnny O'Neal, who provided invaluable editing help with the manuscript.

Raf wishes to thank all of the patients who have inspired him to work hard, listen carefully and appreciate their challenges through their stories that he has been privileged to hear. The collaborations of his coauthor and artist have served to make the book a pleasure to develop. His wife, Jackie has supported him throughout the journey.

Marianne would like to thank Chris and Raf for giving her this opportunity even after she warned them that she had never drawn a cartoon in her life. This book was her first true taste of what her future has in store for her. Of course, she'd also like to thank her parents and her brother for motivating her and being her own personal art critics.

Foreword
by Christian and Liam Lillis
Co-founders of the Peggy Lillis Memorial Foundation

Clostridium difficile (C. diff) is among the most dangerous and least known public health threats facing the United States today. In an era when many of the better-known healthcare-associated infections are decreasing, such as methicillin-resistant *Staphylococcus aureus* (MRSA), pneumonia, and central-line associated blood infections, C. diff is on the rise. In fact, the Centers for Disease Control and Prevention estimate that half a million Americans will be diagnosed with a C. diff infection this year.

From the time of its discovery nearly 50 years ago, C. diff was largely considered a disease of the old and infirm, an infection linked with nursing homes, where it often sickened but rarely killed. That pigeonhole has limited public awareness. Today, most Americans first learn of the disease upon receiving a diagnosis affecting them or a loved one. That's what set our learning curve in motion.

Our mother, Peggy Lillis, was a 56-year-old Irish-Catholic kindergarten teacher in Brooklyn, New York. Though she would admit to needing to lose a few pounds, she was a healthy, robust, and active mom, educator, and beloved member of her community. In her entire life, she had been hospitalized twice, both times to give birth. Like most any teacher, she could catch the occasional cold, flu or stomach bug from her students. Yet most of the time, she didn't even miss work.

That changed when Mom was prescribed the antibiotic clindamycin. A few days into taking the antibiotic, Mom came down with what appeared to be stomach flu. Less than a week later, she died in a local hospital on April 21, 2010 only 36 hours after being admitted. It was during her stay in the hospital that we first learned of C. diff.

We want to be clear. The vast majority of people who have or will contract a C. diff infection will not suffer Mom's fate. Though cases like our mother's are increasing, they remain statistical outliers. Still, the estimated 300 people who died each day from a C. diff infection is a terrible and preventable toll.

In the weeks following our mother's death, we desperately searched for information to help us understand what happened to her. All we could find was written for doctors and researchers by doctors and researchers. There was very little accessible information written with a patient focus.

We also learned of four other people in our circle of friends and family who died from C. diff-related causes that same spring, including a Brooklyn man in his 60s that had a cabana near ours at the beach club, who was being treated for an otherwise non-lethal cancer; a woman in her 40s who was living with multiple sclerosis; and the mother of dear family friends, the Mulligans, who, while in her 80s was in good shape until she acquired C. diff during a hospital stay. In addition to those who lost their lives to C. diff, we found that we knew other people who, while made very ill, ultimately survived their bout with the bacteria.

That is why we are so pleased that Doctors O'Neal and Rizk have written this book. The dearth of easily understandable knowledge about C. diff for those facing the infection firsthand or those at risk and their families helps to fuel this epidemic. We founded The Peggy Lillis Memorial Foundation to change that. In the year since Mom died, we have informed ourselves and worked to inform others via the foundation's Web site, public service announcement, and other advocacy.

Since launching the foundation, we have encountered so many people who, while surviving their C. diff infections, had their lives change forever. In one case, a woman in her 30s who was working as a model struggled with C. diff for months. Though, she survived, the constant diarrhea and dehydration, along with huge amount of antibiotics, have irreparably damaged her gastrointestinal and nervous systems. We have also heard horrifying stories from women who acquired C. diff after giving birth, and even parents of small children who have been afflicted.

We laud the efforts of volunteers, like those who run the online C. diff discussion forum, and those healthcare workers who are on the frontlines of this epidemic every single day, but only a shift in policy will truly address the root causes of this epidemic. Among the policy changes the foundation works toward are stricter antibiotic steward-ship policies. Few guidelines exist for appropriate use of antibiotics, and they are often prescribed unnecessarily. In fact, 20 to 30 percent of antibiotic prescriptions are written for the common cold, a virus, for which they are completely ineffective. This misuse harms not only the person taking a drug unnecessarily, but also the entire community by lessening the drug's effectiveness.

Another area of focus is making C. diff a reportable disease. Currently, only California requires incidences of C. diff infections to be reported to the state, and that law is less than a year old. In order to effectively combat any infectious disease, public health workers must first know where there are outbreaks, the populations that are being afflicted, and how the disease is trending. Without a reportability law, the vast majority of C. diff infections—including those that are fatal—are not recorded. Public health officials and scientists lack the most basic statistics necessary to spot emerging trends, changes in patient populations, and increases in mortality and morbidity.

Policy changes only come when enough people know the damage that C. diff inflicts. That is why educating healthcare workers and consumers is the first step in minimizing death and disability. This book is a critical part of that educational work. While many healthcare workers have heard of C. diff, the general public remains mostly in the dark. As with HIV and tuberculosis, an educated and informed public is key to prevention. There are a great many compassionate doctors and scientists working to ameliorate the damage C. diff causes. But they cannot do it alone. Ordinary Americans, as healthcare consumers, need to demand better reporting and more thorough prevention measures.

Our mother believed deeply in education as a powerful force to create change. That's why we are happy to be working with Doctors O'Neal and Rizk to educate the public and raise awareness of this growing public health threat. We hope you find the book accessible and useful in your or your loved one's recovery from C. diff. To help educate others, we also hope you will use your experience, the information in this book, and the tools The Peggy Lillis Memorial Foundation is providing at www.fightcdiff.org.

We wish you the best in your recovery.

Sincerely,

Christian John Lillis & Liam Lillis
Co-founders, The Peggy Lillis Memorial Foundation

Preface

Three Stories

Desmond, a 37-year-old man, went to the dentist to have a root canal done. To ward off a possible infection, the dentist prescribed Desmond a three-day course of a general antibiotic, beginning on the day of the procedure. The root canal went off without a hitch, but two weeks later Desmond began to have frequent, watery and mucousy diarrhea, accompanied by stomach pain. He assumed it was a case of food poisoning and decided to wait it out. Two weeks later, he was still waiting and decided to visit his doctor. It took another week of tests before Desmond's doctor called to tell Desmond he had something called *C. difficile*.

Julie's mother, 86 years old, was hospitalized with a broken hip. Four days into her mother's hospital stay, Julie learned that her mother was taking oral antibiotics to treat a urinary tract infection associated with her catheter. Julie thought nothing of it; her mother was older, but

1

otherwise quite healthy. A day later, she arrived at the hospital to find that her mother had developed frequent, watery, and bloody diarrhea, extreme stomach pain, and a very high fever. Her mother looked dangerously weak. The next two weeks were a blur. Doctors told Julie her mother had acquired a gut infection called *Clostridium difficile,* and they were treating it with antibiotics. Ten days later, Julie received a call at home from a hospital nurse. Her mother was in serious condition. The nurse explained that the infection was paralyzing her mother's colon, and she would die if her colon was not removed. The surgery occurred the next day, but Julie's mother did not survive the procedure.

While neither Julie nor Desmond had ever heard of C. *difficile,* Renee is all too familiar with it. She has been wrestling off and on with C. *difficile* (or C. diff, as she calls it) for the past eight months. She has what her gastroenterologist calls "recurrent C. *difficile,*" and it hasn't gone away. She has tried any number of antibiotics and other medicines. Each time, the diarrhea subsides for a week or two, and then comes roaring back. She is constantly exhausted and in some degree of pain, has lost 30 pounds, and has had to change to a job that requires less hours. Her marriage has suffered due to her husband's frustration with this never-ending disease. Renee is physically and emotionally spent and sees no end in sight.

A Growing Infectious Threat

If you're reading this book, it's probable that one of the stories above sounds painfully familiar. You are likely suffering from C. *difficile* or have a loved one who is suffering from, or has died of, C. *difficile.* You are very likely scared, angry, or at the very least, frustrated by this awful disease, and you're looking for answers. This book is meant to give you some of those answers, and to educate the public about this emerging infectious disease.

We also hope that it will help you realize that you are not alone. Cases of C. diff have been rising steadily since the 1990s (following Renee's lead above, we will generally refer to *C. difficile* as "C. diff" throughout this book). U.S. hospital discharges for which *Clostridium difficile*–associated disease was listed as any diagnosis almost tripled from 31 per 100,000 members of the population in the 1990s to 84 per 100,000 in 2005[1] and some of the bolder estimates of C. diff infection suggest that up to three million people per year are infected in the U.S. alone[2]. C. diff is not just an American problem; there were 51,681 reports of C. diff disease in elderly Britons in 2006 alone[3], and in one Canadian province, C. diff rates increased from 35.6 cases per 100,000 in 1991 to 156.3 per 100,000 in 2003[4]. In 2008 the Association for Professionals in Infection Control and Epidemiology (APIC) conducted a large scale survey which estimated that 13 out of every 1,000 U.S. hospital patients on any given day were infected or colonized with C. diff[5] (we'll talk about the difference between infected and colonized later), and these numbers may be conservative since C. diff can be widely under-reported.

Frighteningly, C. diff deaths are on the rise as well. In England, there were 499 deaths attributable to C. diff in 1999. In 2006, that number had risen to 3,393. Comparable trends have been seen in the U.S., where *C. difficile*-associated mortality rose from 5.7 per million population in 1999 to 23.7 per million in 2004[6].

The pain of C. diff is financial as well as physical and emotional. The 2008 APIC study estimated that C. diff costs the U.S. health system between $17.6 million and $51.5 million every day! Another study put the number at $3.2 billion per year[7], and these numbers don't take into account health care costs outside of the hospital or nursing home, such as lost productivity and the time that medical professionals must spend treating debilitated patients[8].

Both of the authors of this book are intimately familiar with C. diff. One is a Ph.D. in Biology who, along with his wife, has suffered through multiple bouts with the disease. The other is a gastroenterologist who has treated patients with C. diff since 1993. We know how horrible it can be, and we know how frightening it can be. In this book we'll walk you through our understanding of C. diff, and talk about diagnosing this disease, treating it, and if necessary, living with it. While C. diff does rarely kill some people, the vast majority get over it quickly, and our primary message here is one of hope and optimism. C. diff can be cured, and most often is. When standard treatments don't work, or the bug returns (something we'll talk about extensively in Chapter 3), there are other existing treatment options, and a host of new and promising treatments coming online.

C. diff fact: Look for this little book to provide some answers to your all C. diff questions.

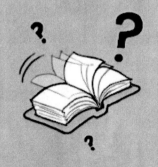

Beating The Beast: How to Use this Book

Patients on the forums at *www.cdiffsupport. com* (a wonderful resource we can't say enough about) call C. diff "The Beast." Our hope is that this book helps you "beat The

Beast," and that it reduces your anxiety and sense of helplessness while doing so.

Fortunately, we are in the middle of an explosion of discovery in C. diff research. To help you digest all of this information, we've annotated the text with some helpful sidebars of C. diff facts, photos, diagrams, explanations of "doctor-speak," "worry boxes" to address the most common C. diff anxieties, and success stories to give you hope.

Doctor-speak: Throughout the text you'll find Doctor-speak boxes like this one that will translate some of the complicated terms doctors use into language we can all understand. Look for these two chatty docs to clue you in.

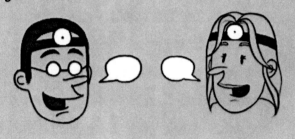

This book is aimed primarily at patients. Whenever possible, we avoid using medical jargon, and try to explain the disease in terms anyone can understand. Because you may want to learn more about

Success Stories: When a patient is in the middle of a C. diff infection, it can feel like it's going to last forever. These success story boxes will present the inspiring stories of C. diff sufferers who fought back against their disease, didn't give up and eventually persevered. Unlike the example stories at the beginning of this preface, these stories are from real patients. Keep in mind that these stories represent C. diff at its worst. Don't assume you're going to have the same experiences these patients did. Instead, take heart that even C. diff at it's worst is beatable!

different aspects of C. diff, we've included endnotes for each chapter that cite the relevant research. Most of this research is written for a medical audience, but it is worth exploring if you are interested. We also hope that this book, and the cited references, will be useful to family and general care practitioners who can find the diagnosis and treatment of C. diff vexing and elusive. We encourage you to share it with your doctor if you have been diagnosed with C. diff.

Worry box: We know C. diff is scary, and sometimes the anxiety it creates can dominate our thinking. Worry boxes like this will address the most common C. diff anxieties and get you to focus on the facts.

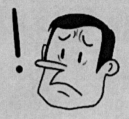

The Legal Stuff

Finally, we must make the point that this book is meant to educate you on the risks of C. diff, the steps your doctor will take to diagnose and treat it, and the research behind that treatment. We also hope it will facilitate a more informed discussion about C. diff between you and your doctor. This book is NOT meant to replace your doctor, and should by no means be used as a tool for self-diagnosis or self-treatment. Additionally, in cases where your doctor and this book seem to disagree, we encourage you to talk more about it with your physician and with other physicians. This book knows nothing about the specifics of your case, and should NOT be seen as a "second opinion." Please don't use it as one.

Notes – Preface

1.   Kelly, C., & LaMont, J. (2008). Clostridium difficle - More difficult than ever. *The New England Journal of Medicine, 359*: 1932.

2.   Parker-Pope, T. (2009, April 14). Stomach bug crystallizes an antibiotic threat. *The New York Times*, p. D1.

3.   Monaghan, T., Boswell, T., & Mahida, Y. (2008). Recent advances in *Clostridium difficile*-associated disease. *Gut, 57*: 850.

4.   Halsey, J. (2008). Current and future treatment modalities for *Clostridium difficile*-associated disease. *American Journal of Health System Pharmacists, 65*: 706.

5.   Association for Professionals in Infection Control and Epidemiology. (2008). National Prevalence Study of *Clostridium difficile* in U.S. Healthcare Facilities. Washington, D.C.: APIC.

6.   Simor, A.E. (2010). Diagnosis, management, and prevention of *Clostridium difficile* infection in long-term care facilities: A review. *Journal of the American Geriatrics Society, 58*: 1556.

7.   O'Brien, J., Lahue, B., Caro, J., & Davidson, D. (2007). The emerging infectious challenge of *Clostridium difficile*-associated disease in Massachusetts hospitals: *Clinical and economic consequences. Infection Control and Hospital Epidemiology , 28* (11): 1223.

8.   DuPont, H.L. (2011). The search for effective treatment for Clostridium difficile infection. *The New England Journal of Medicine, 364*:473.

Chapter One
The Nature of the Beast

One day in June of 2008, Chris, one of the authors of this book, got an anxious call from his wife, Victoria. His normally healthy spouse had been suffering from diarrhea and stomach cramps for the better part of three weeks. Repeated tests for bacteria and parasites had revealed nothing. Looking for answers, their doctor had ordered a series of tests that would not normally be considered for an otherwise healthy young woman who hadn't been in a hospital in months.

"It's something called C. *difficile*," Victoria whispered into the phone. She was very scared. "The doctor said that it can be deadly, and we have to cancel our vacation and stay near a major hospital until the antibiotics kill it."

Despite having a Ph.D. in biology, Chris had never heard of C. diff, or *Clostridium difficile* as it was more properly known. Frightened and surprised, he called their doctor to confirm what his wife had said. Yes, it was serious. Yes, it needed to be treated with antibiotics. Yes, she needed to be careful about spreading it to him and their new baby. And no, the doctor couldn't give much more advice than that.

The next few days were filled with pulse-pounding searches of the Internet and phone calls to knowledgeable friends. Phrases like "toxic megacolon," "multiply recurrent C. difficile," and "pseudomembranous colitis" left them constantly on edge. Every bowel movement called for an examination of the resultant stool. Every bit of stomach pain was cause for alarm. When the first round of C. diff went away, only to come back ten days later, they got even more frightened. When, in the same week, Chris got it as well, they became terrified that their infant daughter could get it. They felt horribly vulnerable, victimized by an infection that didn't seem to obey the normal rules of medical treatment. An online community of fellow sufferers helped, but finding a good doctor and self-education were ultimately the best routes to getting back on track emotionally and physically. Chris and his wife started asking the questions that put them back in control of their illness, and the first question they asked was, "What is this nasty thing called C. diff?"

What is C. diff?

C. diff is a bacteria, one of what we used to call "germs." Its full scientific name is *Clostridium difficile*. Clostridium bacteria like C. diff are big (for germs), rod-shaped bacteria that prefer to live in places without much oxygen. Most commonly, that's deep down in the soil, where they play the very important role of helping to break down dead organic material.

Unfortunately, Clostridium bacteria are also able to live in parts of our intestines, where they can wreak no end of havoc. While you may never have heard of C. diff before you had cause to buy this book, you've likely heard of its infamous cousins: *Clostridium botulinum* and *Clostridium tetani*, which cause botulism and tetanus, respectively. Not all Clostridium bacteria are pathogenic, but many of them, including C. diff, specialize in making toxins that attack and damage the humans and animals they infect. Most pathogenic strains of C. diff produce two toxins. Toxin A disrupts the ability of the intestinal lining to hold together and function properly, while Toxin B enters the cells of the intestinal lining and actively kills them off[1].

The one feature that distinguishes all Clostridium bacteria, and

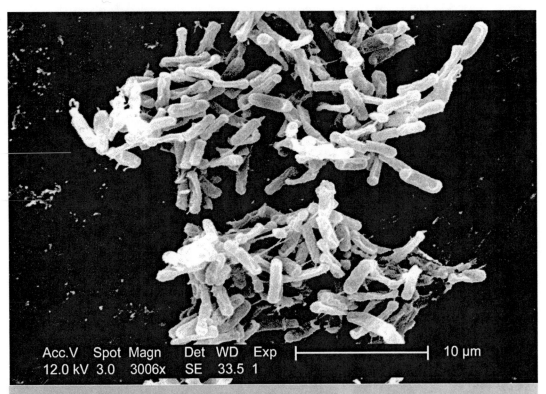

Figure 1.1: A scanning electron micrograph of C. difficile bacteria. Photo courtesy of the CDC. Photo credit: Janice Carr.

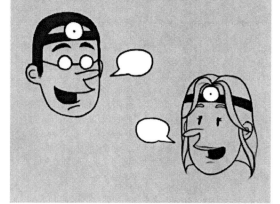

Pathogenic is a big word that simply means "able to cause disease." A pathogenic bacterium is one that is capable of causing harm to humans.

makes them particularly tough to eradicate, is their ability to form "spores." The "vegetative" or active form of C. diff bacteria is pretty fragile – it can live for only about 6 hours on countertops and is easily killed by cleaning agents or stomach acid[2]. But when times get tough for Clostridium bacteria (like when they are exposed to air, or under attack by other bacteria, or even antibiotics) they turn from

their active state to their spore state. As spores, they shut down all unnecessary physiology and grow a hard shell that's impervious to outside dangers, including antibiotics. It's sort of like a snail retreating into its shell at the first sign of trouble, but unlike a snail, these spores can last for five months or more on our countertops, light switches, and faucet handles, doing nothing but waiting for some poor soul to transfer them from hand to mouth and back into the nutrient-rich environments of our guts, where they can morph back into active, toxin-producing bacteria[3]. C. diff is a one-trick pony, but this one trick of making spores causes its victims no end of grief, as we'll see in the pages to come.

C. diff is a diarrheal illness, meaning simply that the primary symptom of infection is diarrhea. Because of that fact, this book is going to talk a lot about what comes out your back end: stool, poop, caca, turds, et cetera. If reading and talking about your stool (an all-inclusive term that we'll use most often) disgusts or embarrasses you, it's time to get over that. Your stool actually has a lot to tell your doctor, but you're going to have to do the talking for it. So sit back, get the chuckles out of your system, and let's take a moment to get the straight poop on your stool.

The Straight Poop

Doctors have recognized for years that there are about seven different stool shapes and patterns. In 1997, some doctors at the University of Bristol in England created a system for categorizing the different stool types to help doctors and patients talk about their stool[4]; they called it the "Bristol Stool Scale"; see our version of it in Figure 1.3.

The doctors from Bristol observed that the main determinant of stool type was the length of time it took food to pass through someone's gut. As stool passes through your large intestine, water is removed from the waste and returned to your blood stream. When stool takes a long time to pass through the large intestine, too much water is taken out of the stool and it becomes hard and pebble-like [Type 1 stools]. If your body can keep just a little water in the stool, you still get a hard stool, but with cracks [Type 2], which is a little easier to push out of the rectum than those darn pebbles that seem to never want to leave. Most agree that the ideal stool is a Type 3 or a Type 4: a log-shaped stool that is smooth and passes with little effort as one piece. On the flip side of the scale, if food moves too quickly through the gut, not enough water is taken out and we get the soft nuggets or mushy applesauce stools that take no effort to empty: a Type 5 or 6. And if your large intestine does not remove enough water from your stool, or adds water back into the stool due to inflammation (as occurs during a C. diff infection), then the result is the dreaded Type 7 stools: watery diarrhea that just gushes out uncontrollably or wakes you up in

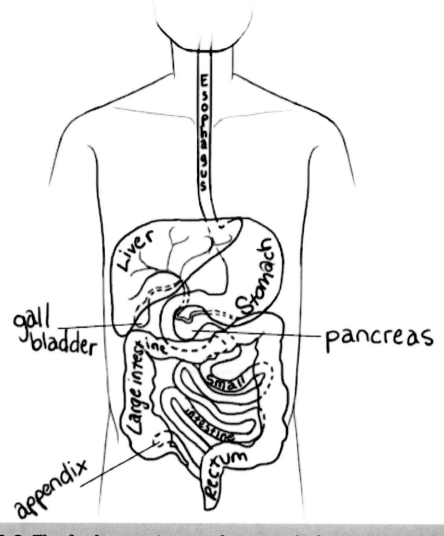

Figure 1.2: The food you eat goes a long way before it sees the light of day again. Food is ingested at the mouth, then passes down the esophagus to the stomach, where stomach acids and enzymes digest it into bits our intestines can absorb. Food leaves the stomach and enters the small intestine, where digestion continues and absorption of nutrients begins. After spending a few hours in the small intestine, the less digestible remains of our meal enter the large intestine, or colon, where bacteria continue to break down hard-to-digest foods, and absorption of water and nutrients is completed. Once everything useful has been removed from the food, it is shipped to the rectum until it's passed as stool from the anus. In a healthy human, it takes an average of 24 to 48 hours for a meal to make the trip from mouth to anus; the biggest determinant of "transit time" is the amount of fiber in the food. High-fiber foods travel more quickly; low-fiber foods travel more slowly.

the middle of the night. Unless you suffer from a chronic gut dysfunction like Irritable Bowel Syndrome, Type 7 stools are your body's way of telling you, "Something's wrong down here!"

It is important to know that even during healthy times, the shape, feel, and color of stool can vary quite a bit. We can be disease-free and still have really bad looking watery stool that flip flops in the next bowel movement to hard stools. Gut transit time, and the resulting stools, can vary a

BRISTOL STOOL CHART

Type		Description
1		Tiny, hard lumps that are very difficult to pass
2		Sausage-shaped, but clearly made of distinct lumps
3		Sausage-shaped with visible cracks in the surface
4		Snake-like, smooth, and soft
5		Soft blobs that are easily passed
6		Fluffy, ragged pieces; pudding-like
7		Watery with no solid pieces

Figure 1.3: The Bristol Stool Scale: the definitive guide to talking about your poop.

lot and most often varies because of daily changes in your diet. High fiber foods tend to move more quickly through the gut, while lower fiber foods tend to stay in the gut a bit longer. You'll need to keep this in mind in Chapter 4, when we talk about what happens after you've killed off your C. diff infection, and your guts are trying to get back to perfect health.

An individual's stool also changes color a lot. Doctors consider varying shades of brown, green, and yellow stool to be normal and largely dependent on what people haveeaten, or on the medications they are taking. There are two colors of stool to pay attention to that generally mean illness and need medical evaluation: black and varying shades of red. Black stool, especially if it is sticky and shiny, will almost always mean there is blood in the stool coming from somewhere in the stomach or small intestine. Medications can also cause black stool, notably: iron supplements, Pepto Bismol, and Kaopectate. When stool appears red (like strawberries or lipstick) or dark red, the source of blood is likely closer to the anus (such as from a hemorrhoid). All types of bloody stool, whether they are solid or liquid, need a thorough medical evaluation. Diarrhea (including C. diff diarrhea) is often, but not always, green. That green color comes from bile, a green-colored diges-

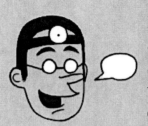

Hemorrhoid: Hemorrhoids are veins inside the rectum (the part of the digestive system just inside the anus) that become inflamed and enlarged due to pressure. This pressure most commonly comes from the straining that comes with passing stools that are too hard. The walls of hemorrhoids are prone to bleeding out surprisingly large amounts of bright red blood. They are annoying, painful, itchy, and depending on how much they bleed, potentially embarrassing, but they are not life threatening.

tive enzyme that's released high in your digestive tract and is normally broken down by the time your stool is excreted. Because diarrhea moves so quickly through your intestines, there's no time to properly break down that bile, and it colors the diarrhea green.

Why Does C. difficile Give Me Diarrhea?

It's probably no surprise to you that patients with C. diff tend to have those dreaded Type 7 diarrheal stools. It's one of the requirements for a C. diff diagnosis, and generally the first sign that something is wrong. However, different people with C. diff will display different symptoms. Some will have mild diarrhea that is easily treated and stopped. Others will have more severe symptoms like extreme urgency to defecate (urgent enough to wake them up at night), profuse watery, unformed, and sometimes bloody diarrhea; fever; high white blood cell counts; tiredness; pain; and very tender tummies[5].

Most of these symptoms arise from the way C. diff colonizes and infects the gut. C. diff infection often leads to a phenomenon in the large intestine called pseudomembranous colitis. The "pseudomembranes" part of this refers to the membranous spots that C. diff creates on the wall of the large intestine as it settles in to do damage; imagine

What's that smell? For some reason, many C. diff sites on the Web mention the distinct and awful odor that C. diff diarrhea has. It has been described as rotting meat, manure-like, and even "iron-y." Unless you are a health-care professional with daily experience with the smell, we don't recommend doing much sniffing of your stool. The odor of stool varies with what is eaten, what is not digested and what the person normally produces for gas from fermentation of undigested foods in the colon. So odor can change on a day-to-day basis. Diarrhea smells differently from normal stool for a number of reasons. Just because you've "never smelled that smell before" doesn't necessarily mean you have C. diff. We'll get into diagnosis in the next chapter and talk about more reliable ways your doctor can diagnose your diarrhea.

hundreds of big, inflamed scabs on the walls of your guts. The "colitis" part refers to the inflammation and damage to the colon that results from the toxins A and B described above. There are a few other causes of pseudomembranous colitis, but C. diff is by far the most common[6].

At the microscopic level, the toxins that C. diff produces are actually poisoning the cells that make up the large intestine. As these cells become sicker and sicker, more and more of them die and stop performing their intended function: pulling nutrients, minerals, and water out of the food that your stomach and small intestine have processed. If the colon can't do its job of recovering that water, the C. diff patient can rapidly dehydrate and lose minerals essential to healthy living. If the diarrhea is bad enough, and the resulting dehydration is bad enough, lots of other bodily functions will start to suffer. In most cases, it is this dehydration which poses the greatest risk to the C. diff patient.

For a very unlucky minority, C. diff will progress beyond the "severe" stage and result in symptoms that are immediately life threatening. If C. diff is left untreated long enough, or does not respond to initial treatments, the poisons it produces may lead to a poorly understood

Diarrhea is good? Diarrhea is a scary phenomenon, and not something we want to have for long, but it's important to remember that diarrhea serves a valuable function in our body: the quicker our guts can empty, the less time harmful bacteria spend in them. So, from one perspective, diarrhea is helpful in cleaning out the bad bugs making us sick. C. diff diarrhea, unfortunately, just lasts too long to be healthy.

phenomenon called toxic megacolon in which the C. diff toxins horribly damage the patient's large intestine, necessitating extreme measures and even surgery to save the patient's life. The risk of death from C. diff is small but real. Approximately 1.5-2% of patients who are hospitalized for C. diff will die from it[7]. However, because there are so many patients who get C. diff, that 1.5-2% can add up to a lot of deaths, between 30,000 and 100,000 yearly depending on the source of the estimate (because C. diff patients often have other complications, it's very difficult to be certain that the cause of death was their C. diff).

How Do People Get C. diff?

C. diff infections are passed from one person to another through what doctors call the fecal-oral route. To put it delicately, C. diff exits one victim's body during a bowel movement and then makes its way to another victim's mouth (usually by contamination of hands), where it is ingested, and makes its way down into the second victim's gut. This is not as uncommon an event as you might think. Even the best hand washers are likely ingesting thousands, if not hundreds of thousands of bacteria every day. Many of these bacteria are harmless, or even helpful to us, but some are pathogenic. The vast majority of these harmful bacteria are killed in the stomach by our stomach acid and never make it down to the warm,

Hospital-acquired Infection: Doctors call C. diff a hospital-acquired infection. This is just a very fancy way of saying "an illness that developed during (or due to) hospitalization or treatment."

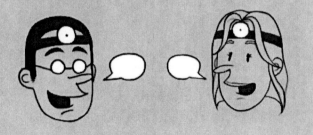

18

Confusing "Can Happen" With "Will Happen:" If your heart rate is up and your worry factor is through the roof as you've read these last few pages, then it's time to put things in perspective. First, please know that almost all C. diff deaths occur in very old and frail patients, or those with other life-threatening diseases. If you have the strength to read this book, and you have C. diff, the odds that it will kill you are very, very low, especially if you are under the care of a doctor and are aware of your own symptoms. Can we give you an iron-clad guarantee that C. diff won't kill you? No, no more than we can give you a guarantee that you won't be killed in a car accident on your way to work tomorrow. For the moment, take a deep breath, relax, and throw up a big red stop sign in your head if you find yourself starting to obsess about very unlikely things.

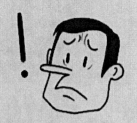

wet, nutrient-rich bacterial paradise we call our small and large intestines. Unfortunately, that same trick of forming spores that makes C. diff capable of surviving for months on your countertops also makes it more resistant to stomach acid, increasing the chance that ingested C. diff spores will make it down into the gut, where they will get comfortable and revert back into live C. diff bacteria.

So why doesn't everyone have C. diff? Well, the stomach isn't our last line of defense. Even if a pathogenic bacterium like C. diff does make it all the way down to our guts, it then has to compete with the millions of good, friendly bacteria that happily live there, helping us fully digest our food and forming the bulk of our gut's immune system.

Imagine your gut is a lush field of grass, and the bacteria in it are a giant herd of cows (billions and billions of cows) feeding on every available inch of that grass (in this metaphor, the food we ingest and pass through our guts is the grass). In this field, there's just not enough room to add another cow; the competition for resources in our gut makes it very difficult for foreign bacteria to get established, and C. diff is generally a pretty wimpy bacterium; it does a very poor job of competing with the resident bacteria in our gut. So, if a healthy person with a healthy gut flora ingests a little C. diff, it's generally no big deal — the C. diff just can't get enough of a foothold amidst all the other bacteria to cause any problems. In fact, we know from testing that a small portion of the adult population have pathogenic C. diff permanently living inside them in small numbers. These carriers can spread C. diff to others, but as long as they maintain a healthy gut flora, they'll never have any problems themselves.

Carriers: Interestingly enough, lots of people carry C. diff around harmlessly, never suffering any symptoms. This includes up to 5% of the non-hospitalized adult population and up to 60% of newborns! In one hospital study, 20% of newly admitted patients tested positive for C. diff, but two-thirds of these patients never developed the symptoms of C. diff[8]. Carrying C. difficile without showing any symptoms may actually indicate that you have some natural resistance to C. diff infection and are less likely to develop C. diff diarrhea. Another hospital study found that only 1% of those already colonized on admittance developed C. diff symptoms, while 3.6% of those not colonized eventually developed C. diff and C. diff symptoms. This is a small but statistically significant difference[9].

So if C. diff is such a wimpy little bug, how does it get to be such a big problem for so many people? Remember that one trick of forming spores? Yep, once again it's the secret to C. diff's success.

Once C. diff makes it way through the high acid environment of the stomach, it will gradually make it's way down to the "oh-so-perfect" environment of our large intestine. It is now faced with a decision: Should it try to get established, or should it instead remain a nice, hardy spore and wait for better times? If a person's gut flora is healthy and robust, C. diff will always opt for the latter. Better to sit as a spore for a while doing nothing than try to make it as an active bacterium and get jostled and mobbed by the other bacteria of the gut flora. What is C. diff waiting for? It's waiting for some disturbance that clears out the resident gut flora and creates an opportunity for growth. Let's go back to our cow and field metaphor (check out Figure 1.6). Imagine our giant herd of a billion cows was suddenly reduced down to ten or twelve cows. Sud-

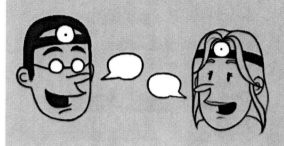

Flora is a fancy word to describe the amount and variety of bacteria in our guts.

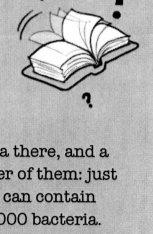

Billions and billions: The amount and variety of bacteria in a healthy gut is pretty amazing. There are over 500 species of bacteria there, and a staggering number of them: just one gram of stool can contain 10,000,000,000,000 bacteria. We're not even sure what the word is for that many zeros...quadrillions? Anyway, it's a lot.

denly our invader cow is looking at a wide-open field of delectable grass. He's going to go hog (or cow) wild. This reduction in friendly gut flora is generally the trigger that sets a C. diff infection off, and in modern times, this gut disturbance most often comes in the form of broad spectrum antibiotics.

The Double-Edged Sword Of Antibiotics

Starting with the discovery of penicillin in 1928, antibiotics have revolutionized health care and saved hundreds of thousands of lives. While some antibiotics are quite specific, and can be targeted to kill only the type of bacterium that a doctor is interested in killing, others kill many different kinds of bacteria. This is where our problems begin.

Let's imagine a patient goes to the emergency room for what turns out to be a urinary tract infection, one of the more common infections seen in hospitals. The doctor who sees the patient will undoubtedly give the patient an oral antibiotic for this infection. In most cases, this treatment will work wonders: The infection will clear up, and the patient will enjoy the fruits of modern medicine. But in some cases, the antibiotic will kill the bacteria causing the urinary tract infection *and* also attack much of the other bacteria in the patient's

Figure 1.4 (facing page): Most of the time, when C. diff bacteria make it into our guts, they're jostling and shoving like one cow in a giant herd of cows, all fighting over limited pasture land. But when antibiotics start to whittle down the size of the "herd," C. diff spores hide out and don't get killed by the antibiotics. This means that once the antibiotics have stopped, and that giant herd of competing gut bacteria are gone, C. diff starts to reproduce like crazy in that wide-open field that is our recently-medicated guts. Pretty soon, the herd isn't looking so friendly anymore; it's all C. diff.

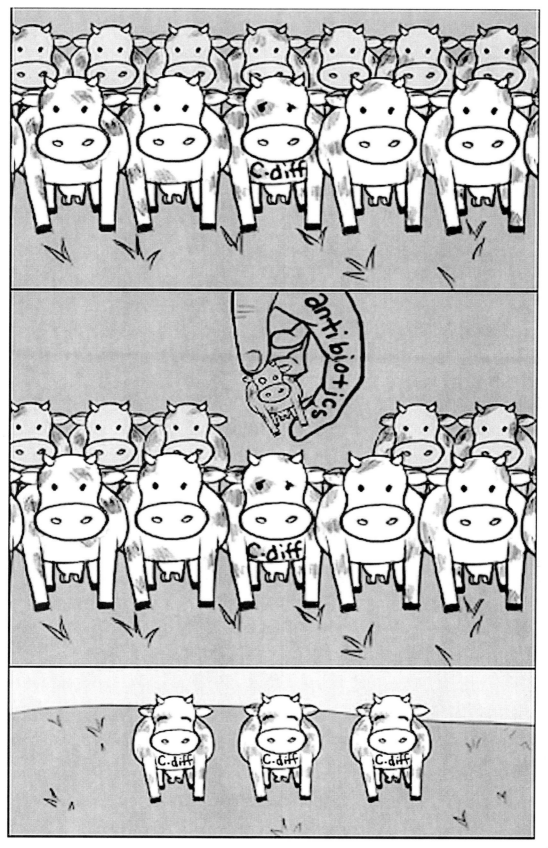

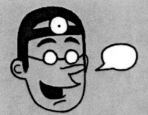

Strains: Different "strains" of bacteria are like different breeds of dogs. Genetically they are the same species but differ slightly in appearance, where they prefer to live, and other characteristics. There are over 400 known strains of C. difficile bacteria, and not all of them are pathogenic!

body, including those that keep the gut healthy and functioning. If this happens, and the patient happens to ingest C. diff spores at the same time, the patient may be heading for a C. diff infection. This sort of event is called antibiotic-associated diarrhea (or AAD), and about 20%-50% of all antibiotic-associated diarrhea is due to C. diff spores sprouting and taking over in a patient's now vulnerable gut[10]. We should also note that many strains of C. diff bacteria have developed resistance to certain antibiotics (most notably what doctors call fluoro-quinolones); this is another reason that giving antibiotics can cause C. diff -- depending on the type of antibiotic, it may kill everything but the C. diff[11]!

Perhaps the most common place to receive antibiotics is in the hospital. Unfortunately, hospitals and long-term care facilities are literally covered in C. diff[12], and it is all too simple for a doctor or other health care provider to transfer C. diff from one patient to another. This unfortunate double whammy of antibiotics and high C. diff infestation leads to some pretty astonishing and scary statistics. In one study, 13% of patients in the hospital for more than one week were colonized with C. diff. This number increased to 50% for those in the hospital more than four weeks[13]. Colonization in long-term care facilities is much lower,

How Long Will Antibiotics Make Me Susceptible To C. Diff? Most C. diff infections make themselves known within a day to four weeks after antibiotic usage. However, antibiotics may lead to a disruption of the intestinal flora and resultant C. diff infection up to three months or more after usage[16]! Still, it's important to remember that every day that passes after taking antibiotics lessens your chances of getting C. diff.

about 5%-7%[14]. We can compare these numbers to the 5% of the normal, healthy population that is colonized with C. diff, and conclude that the best place to get C. diff is, unfortunately, the hospital. This conclusion is further supported when we look at the low numbers of C. diff acquired out in the community: only 7.7 cases per 100,000 people per year of observation in 1998[15]. That is very, very low.

Up to this point we've established that if patients experience a disruption of their normal gut bacteria and are simultaneously exposed to C. diff bacteria, they are at risk for an infection. But we've left out one important factor: the patients themselves.

It turns out that not everyone is created equal when it comes to C. diff resistance. Some patients seem to be more resistant to C. diff than others. We've already

Not all diarrhea is C. diff: The fact that only about 20%-50% of antibiotic-associated diarrhea is attributable to C. diff sends an important message to doctors and patients. It means that while C. diff should always be suspected if a patient gets diarrhea after antibiotic use, it should not be assumed.

Figure 1.5 (Facing Page): Figure 1.5 illustrates how exposure to C. diff and some gut flora disruption, like antibiotics, can lead to three possible clinical outcomes. Jim, who already has C. diff antibodies in his system, has no negative reaction to C. diff. He just carries the bacteria around for a while without even knowing it. Tim doesn't have C. diff antibodies but is capable of making them. Tim has an initial episode of illness in response to his C. diff exposure, but recovers quickly with treatment and never has C. diff again. Unlucky Kim doesn't have C. diff antibodies, and her body will never do a good job of making them, regardless of how many times she has C. diff. Kim may recover quickly with treatment, but she may also require multiple rounds of treatment to handle what has become recurrent C. diff. Kim's immune system isn't going to help her out on this one much; she'll have to rely on antibiotics and the recovery of her own gut flora if she wants to get better. If you're suffering through recurrent C. diff now, chances are good that you're a "Kim."

learned that the elderly and infirm are more likely to develop C. diff than younger, healthier patents, but there may be a genetic difference as well. A number of studies have demonstrated that some patients mount a stronger immune system response to C. diff toxins than others. Not surprisingly, those patients with a stronger immune response seem less likely to get C. diff diarrhea, and are somewhat less likely to have recurrent C. diff[17]. This is a disappointing finding for those patients who don't mount a strong immune response to C. diff, but holds out some tantalizing possibilities for the success of vaccines in preventing and treating C. diff. More on that in Chapter 5.

One final word here on acquiring a C. diff infection, and it is an important one: The vast majority of patients who are given antibiotics will never develop a C. diff infection. To put some numbers behind this, in 1994, there were only 6.7 cases of C. diff per 100,000 exposures to

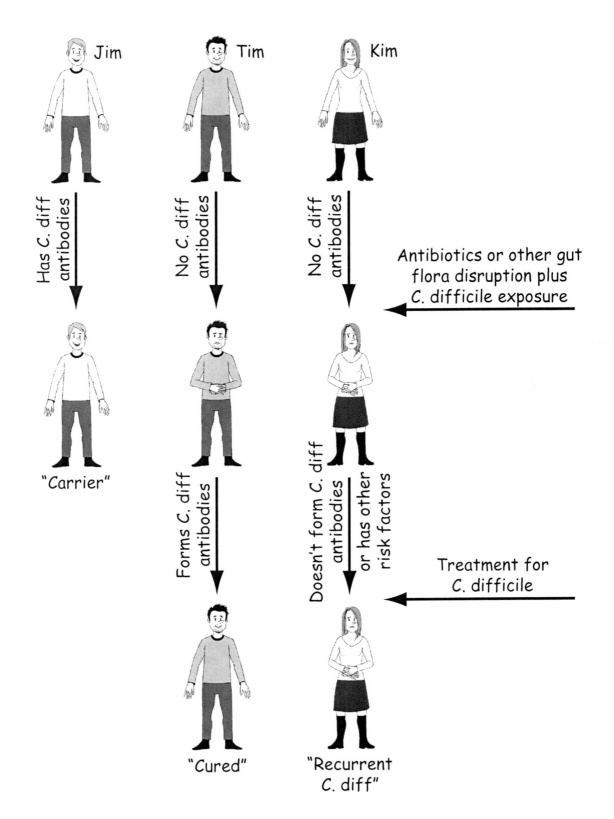

Not all antibiotics are equally likely to result in C. diff: The worst offenders are the broad-spectrum antibiotics that kill all bacteria in the body, good or bad. These include some penicillins, cephalosporins, and clindamycin. It also seems that taking multiple antibiotics at once may be more likely to result in C. diff infection[18]. See Table 1.1 for a complete listing of safer and less safe antibiotics.

antibiotics[19]. While this number has grown over the years by a sizeable amount, antibiotic use still remains very, very safe. Why is this? C. diff researchers describe a "three hit rule" for C. diff infection. They suggest that two components appear to be essential for C. diff infection: 1) exposure to antibiotics (or other inciting incident), and 2) exposure to toxic C. diff. They note that even with these two components, most of the exposed and endangered will still not develop C. diff. They think that one additional factor is necessary for an "infection" of C. diff to occur. They note that this "third hit" could be related to the patient's susceptibility to infection, or the virulence of their particular C. diff strain, or even the type and timing of the antibiotics they received.

Preventing C. diff

If you're reading this book, chances are the advice here on preventing C. diff is too little and too late for you. However, in the interest of avoiding both future infections and the spread of C. diff to others, let's talk a little bit about measures to prevent C. diff infection.

A 1997 report from the American College of Gastroenterology[20] presented a number of measures for preventing the spread of C. diff.

We summarize them here:

Avoid Antibiotics

In a 2008 survey of C. diff infections in hospitals, 79.4% of C. diff-infected patients had received antibiotics before the onset of their disease[21]. Without a doubt, avoiding antibiotics (when prudent) goes a long way in preventing C. diff infections. One study restricting clindamycin (a common broad-spectrum antibiotic) use in hospitals dropped the rate of C. diff infections from 22.5 per 1,000 discharges to 7.4 per 1,000 discharges over a one year period[22]. However, we feel

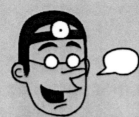

Colonization vs. Infection: It is important to remember that colonization does not equal infection. Many people are colonized with C. diff, meaning only that they carry it for some period of time, without ever showing symptoms of an infection. This is one of the reasons that doctors rarely test to see if they've cured someone of C. diff. Many patients will continue to test positive for C. diff long after they stop having C. diff symptoms. These patients are still "colonized" by the bacterium, but aren't "infected" with it.

we must say here that in general, when used prudently, antibiotics are a good thing – perhaps the best thing to happen to medicine...ever! Although many antibiotics are prescribed unnecessarily (as much as 30% by some estimates), we encourage you not to say no to antibiotics that you really need. There is no point in getting gravely ill from one infection just to avoid the possibility of another. In table 1.1, we present a classification of antibiotics by their relative risk of causing C. diff.

Keep in mind that any antibiotic, no matter how safe, carries with it a risk of C. diff infection.

Avoid Gastric Acid-Suppressing Medications

There is more and more evidence that a class of medicines called proton pump inhibitors (marketed as Nexium, Prilosec, and Prevacid) may contribute to C. diff. Proton pump inhibitors are prescribed to

I have C. diff and I'm terrified my child is going to get it too! This is an understandable worry, but not as critical a one as you might think. First off, transmission of C. diff between family members is relatively rare unless others in your family are also using antibiotics; this applies to babies and children as well as adults. Secondly, babies, particularly in their first year, rarely 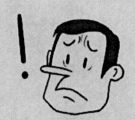 have C. diff symptoms, even though studies have estimated that 40-60% of babies are harmlessly colonized with C. diff[25]. In fact, C. diff was first described in 1935 as a normal part of babies' digestive flora! While this "immunity" to C. diff declines after baby's first year, babies and young children still seem to tolerate C. diff well, even when they get it. No one is quite sure why babies and toddlers are so good at carrying C. diff without suffering from it, but some suggest that the cells of their immature guts don't yet have enough places for C. diff toxins to latch onto[26]. Having said this, C. diff infection does happen in kids (as two of the success stories in this book will attest), and at least one research group has documented an increase in C. diff infections in children and the severity of those infections. If your child develops diarrhea while you or someone else in your family has C. diff, then certainly you are within the realm of "playing it safe" to get their stool tested (but keep in mind that diarrhea due to non-C. diff causes is all too common in children in the first few years of life).

Most likely to Cause C. difficile	More likely to Cause C. difficile	Less Likely to Cause C. difficile
clindamycin	ciprofloxacin	sulfa drugs
cephalixin	levofloxacin	aminoglycosides
cefuroxime	moxifloxacin	metronidazole
cefaclor	cotrmoxazole	vancomycin
moxifoxacin	erythromycin	trimethoprim
ceftazidim	clarithromycin	priptazobactam
imipenem	azithromycin	tetracyclines
cephalosporins	macrolides	
flouroquinolones	nitrofurantoin	
augmentin	amoxicillin	
	ampicillin	

Table 1.1: A classification of popular antibiotics by their C. diff risk. Note that the industry names for drugs are listed here, not the names they are marketed under. Keep in mind that this classification shows relative risk; all antibiotics (including those in the right-most column) carry some risk of precipitating a C. diff infection. Note also that this list is incomplete, and there are numerous other antibiotics on the market with varying degrees of C. diff risk. This list was compiled from numerous sources, some of which differ on how they classify a particular drug's risk. Different authors are likely to disagree on some of these rankings.

reduce heartburn and gastro-esophogeal reflux disease. They do this by reducing the levels of acids in the stomach, which is very helpful for heartburn, but unfortunately this reduces the gut's ability to kill harmful bacteria like C. diff. By at least one estimate, proton pump inhibitors double your risk of a C. diff infection[23]. This is nowhere near the risk posed by antibiotics, but it's worth looking at if you're worried about C.

In 1979, after his pediatrician prescribed amoxicillin for bronchitis and an ear infection, my four-year-old son developed Clostridium difficile. Doctors then knew little about the infection. He was hospitalized, comatose and ill for weeks, and was one of the first patients treated with oral vancomycin. He had two relapses and developed C. diff again in 1985 after taking erythromycin.

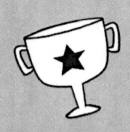

In March 1993, an allergist prescribed a "new" antibiotic, Vantin, to me for sinusitis. I developed C. diff. symptoms, and a gastroenterologist diagnosed pseudomembranous colitis. I was hospitalized with sinusitis, pneumonia, a UTI, and C. diff, put on several antibiotics and had sinus surgery. I ground my teeth from stress, broke two teeth and developed osteomyletis in my jaw. I was on IV and oral vancomycin for seven weeks and had my mouth rebuilt.

In September 1993, I went to a prestigious midwestern clinic. The doctor there diagnosed me with IBS. I disagreed, but all my C. diff tests were negative. I went off vancomycin, became ill, saw a doctor in Kansas City and tested positive – one of my few positive tests. That doctor did a "broth" procedure to install good bacteria in my GI tract by endoscope. It failed. I enrolled in a blind study for S. boulardii (now Florastor) and was on compassionate usage for two years without success. I contacted a doctor who had developed a new probiotic and took it for over a year; it failed.

I had C. diff continuously between 1993-1997 but continued to work. In 1997, my doctor administered "the broth" again; it was successful. In 1999, I was hospitalized with pneumonia, put on Levequin, and developed C. diff again. "The broth" was successful in treating it.

Before C. diff., I was healthy but developed multiple health issues later. Doctors agree it affected my immune system and believe I'm at high risk of developing it again. I spoke before a committee of the Kansas legislature to mandate that C. diff be reported (without success), was featured in a local health magazine, and have moderated a C. diff support site for ten years. I exercise constantly, am in numerous activities, and travel, including a yearly trip to the UK to see my older son and his family. I've beaten C. diff (multiple times), and you can too.

Bobbie Smith, Kansas City

diff, particularly since many of these drugs may be wrongly prescribed or ineffective for what they are prescribed for[24].

Take Probiotics

If you must take antibiotics (your doctor will let you know when the risk of an infection outweighs the risk of developing C. diff), consider taking probiotics along with them. Probiotics are specially prepared "good" bacteria that help replace any bacteria antibiotics might kill in our guts. They come in pill or drink form and are in almost all yogurt. Probiotic organisms serve a number of beneficial functions, including helping us digest our food, altering our intestinal environment to be less favorable for disease-causing microorganisms, enhancing the function of our gut wall, producing chemicals that kill harmful bacteria, and even inducing our immune system to better fight off harmful microorganisms like C. diff.

Probiotics have been successfully used to prevent C. diff infections. One probiotic, a yeast called *Saccharomyces boulardii,* was shown to reduce the rates of C. diff colonization from 31% to 9.4% when given with antibiotics[27]. This remarkable finding has been supported by broader studies as well. Other studies have delivered mixed results on the power of probiotics in helping to prevent C. diff infections after antibiotic use[28], but they seem to offer a chance of reducing rates of C. diff infection with few side effects in otherwise healthy patients.

Wash Your Hands and Use Gloves

Not surprisingly, one of the best ways to stay free of C. diff (and indeed, most infectious diseases) is to regularly wash your hands after

Sanitizing gels not so sanitary: Many doctors and patients favor sanitizing gels over washing with soap because the soap dries out their hands. Unfortunately, antibiotic sanitizing gels do a great job of killing viruses and many bacteria, but they do not kill C. diff spores, which makes them far less effective than hand washing in preventing C. diff transmission[32].

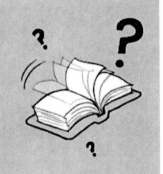

using the bathroom, before preparing food and after contact with others who are ill[29]. This recommendation applies to doctors as well as patients, and you should feel comfortable asking your doctor to wash his or her hands before an examination (or even before shaking hands). One study found C. diff on the hands of nearly 60% of doctors and nurses at one hospital[30]. Glove use works well too. In one study, routine glove use and disposal by doctors at a hospital dropped the rate of C. diff infections from 7.7 per 1,000 discharges to 1.5 per 1,000 discharges[31]. There is some concern that doctors' and nurses' scrubs may be contaminated with C. diff spores and may be one path that C. diff is taking from the hospital into the community. Some authorities are encouraging doctors and nurses not

How long can spores live in the environment? To our knowledge, no one has done a good study looking at how long C. diff spores can live in the environment and still be able to give someone a C. diff infection. There is some general agreement that the length of time is on the order of months, but no one really seems to know an exact number.

Take two aspirin and call me in the morning. Believe it or not, the lowly aspirin may be one of the tools doctors include in their C. diff fighting tool kits someday. Patients taking 81mg of aspirin a day for heart health were 40% less likely to get C. diff than their non-aspirin chugging peers. The reduction in C. diff risk was even greater for those taking higher doses of aspirin[36]. This may be because aspirin changes the pH of the gut to an acidity level that C. diff doesn't like. It may also have something to do with the anti-inflammatory properties of the drug. Talk to your doctor before you start popping aspirin pills, however. Aspirin has long been known to be toxic in large doses (to your ears especially), and may interfere with other medications you are on.

to wear their scrubs outside of the hospital, but don't panic if you see a medical worker out in their "whites" or "greens"; this issue has not been studied very much yet.

Clean Possibly Contaminated Spaces

Regular disinfection of hard surfaces (light switches, door knobs, countertops, toilets, bed posts, etc.) in hospitals results in a significant reduction in C. diff cases. Disinfecting hard surfaces, especially in the bathroom, can also be helpful at home. While hospitals tend to use extra-strong industrial cleaners, a mixture of 1 part sodium hypochlorite bleach to 10 parts water will create a C. diff-killing solution that's perfect for the home bathroom. The clothes of C. diff patients should be washed separately, if possible, and they should use a different bathroom than others in the house, if possible. Again, transmission between family members who haven't been on antibiotics is quite rare, so most of this cleaning is done with the goal of preventing future reinfection in the already ill patient by those pesky spores!

Isolate Patients with C. diff

There is considerable disagreement over whether to isolate patients infected with C. diff. Some authors have reported higher rates of C. diff infection in hospital patients sharing a room with an already infected patient[33], while other studies have found no connection. Certainly, hospital rooms with C. diff patients have more C. diff bacteria and spores contaminating surfaces. Exposure may also be reduced by using disposable instruments, thermometers, etc.[34] However, before you go demanding a private room the next time you are in the hospital, remember that simply being exposed to C. diff is rarely enough to acquire an infection.

The Changing Nature Of C. diff

Up until the last two decades, C. diff was a reliably mundane and uncommon infection. Cases were relatively rare, and those cases that did spring up tended to do so according to the rules outlined above: in hospitals, after antibiotic use, typically in already at-risk patients. Sadly, that is no longer the case.

Public health monitors have observed a frightening increase in C. diff infections in hospitalized children, a group previously thought to be at relative low risk for C. diff. In 1997, there were only 3,565 documented cases of C. diff in hospitalized children. By 2006 that number had risen to 7,779 cases[35], or about a 15% increase in infections each year. More and more cases of community-acquired C. diff are arising. This refers to those cases of C. diff contracted without any hospital stay, and it speaks to the growing prevalence and toxicity of C. diff strains in the environment. Almost half of the C. diff cases in Glasgow, Scotland, in 2010 were contracted out the hospital, and similar findings have been reported elsewhere. Why is this happening? C. diff, even toxic C. diff, is present naturally in the environment, but at least one study suggested that some of the community-acquired cases were infected with strains that originated in the hospital. This suggests that C. diff is "escaping" hospitals, being carried into the community and spreading to others previously not at risk to exposure[37]. We're now also finding C. diff in the foods we eat. At least one study found toxin-producing C. diff in 42% of the meat products sampled from three grocery stores in the southwestern United States[38].

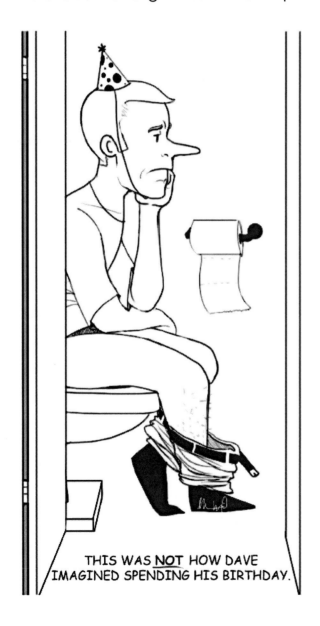

THIS WAS **NOT** HOW DAVE IMAGINED SPENDING HIS BIRTHDAY.

More frightening is the emergence of hypervirulent strains of C. diff. The BI/NAP1 strain is the most famous, most common, and most frightening of these new strains (the complicated name comes from the way in which biologists classify different strains of bacteria). BI/NAP1 has shown resistance to some commonly-used antibiotics (though not the ones used to treat C. diff!) and has a series of genetic mutations that lead to highly increased toxicity compared to non-BI/NAP1 strains of C. diff[39]. This increased toxicity seems to come from much higher production of toxins by this strain, some 16 to 23 times more toxin than is produced by traditionally known strains of C. diff[40]. BI/NAP1 also produces a toxin not previously seen in C. diff called binary toxin. It's unclear what role this binary toxin plays in C. diff illness, but it isn't likely to be good.

This higher level of toxicity leads to more severe infections from this strain and is associated with much higher death rates. In one Canadian hospital that saw an outbreak of BI/NAP1, death rates jumped from 4.7% of patients in 1991-92 to 12.8% of patients in 2003[41]. Other studies have confirmed this doubling of death rates in BI/NAP1 cases. BI/NAP1 has already been implicated in numerous other hospital outbreaks of C. diff in North America and Europe. Fortunately, this nasty strain of C. diff still responds well to the antibiotics typically used to treat C. diff, but it moves more quickly and hits harder than many doctors expect. BI/NAP1 is keeping gastroenterologists and infection disease doctors on their toes, and it should be considered a frightening warning of what other dangerous strains of C. diff may arise in the future.

Notes - Chapter One

1. Lylerly, D.M., Krivan, H.C., & Wilkins, T.D. (1988). *Clostridium difficile*: Its disease and toxins. Clinical Microbiology Reviews, 1: 1.

2. Jump, R.L.P., Pultz, M.J., & Donskey, C.J. (2007). Vegetative *Clostridium difficile* survives in room air on moist surfaces and in gastric contents with reduced acidity: A potential mechanism to explain the association between proton pump inhibitors and *C. difficile*-associated diarrhea? Antimicrobial Agents and Chemotherapy, 51(8): 2883.

3. Hota, B. (2004). Contamination, disinfection, and cross-colonization: Are hospital surfaces reservoirs for nosocomial infection? Clinical Infectious Diseases, 39(8): 1182.

4. Lewis, S.J, & Heaton, K.W. (1997). Stool form scale as a useful guide to intestinal transit time. Scandinavian Journal of Gastroenterology, 32: 920.

5. Kelly, C.P., Pothoulakis, C., & LaMont, J.T. (1994). *Clostridium difficile* colitis. The New England Journal of Medicine, 330: 257.

6. Bartlett, J.G. (2008). Historical perspectives on studies of *Clostridium difficile* and *C. difficile* infection. Clinical Infectious Diseases, 46: S4.

7. Tonna, I, & Welsby, P.D. (2005). Pathogenesis and treatment of *Clostridium difficile* infection. Postgraduate Medical Journal, 81: 367.

8. Gerding, D.N, Johnson, S., Peterson, L.R., Mulligan, M.E., & Silva, Jr., J. (1995). *Clostridium difficile*-associated diarrhea and colitis. Infection Control and Hospital Epidemiology, 16: 459.

9. Poutanen, S.M., & Simor, A.E. (2004). *Clostridium difficile*-associated diarrhea in adults. Canadian Medical Association Journal, 171: 51.

10. Segarra-Newnham, M. (2007). Probiotics for *Clostridium difficile*–Associated Diarrhea: Focus on Lactobacillus rhamnosus GG and Saccharomyces boulardii. The Annals of Pharmacotherapy, 41: 1212.

11. Halsey, J. (2008). Current and future treatment modalities for *Clostridium difficile*-associated disease. American Journal of Health-System Pharmacy, 65: 705.

12. Kelly, Pothoulakis, & LaMont, 1994.

13. Johnson, S. & Gerding, D.N. (1998). *Clostridium difficile*-associated diarrhea. Cliniclal Infectious Diseases, 26: 1027.

14. Poutanen & Simor, 2004.

15. Johnson & Gerding, 1998.

16. McFarland, L.V. (2005). Alternative treatments for *Clostridium difficile* disease: What really works? Journal of Medical Microbiology, 54: 101.

17. Johal, S.S., Lambert, C.P., Hammond, J., James, P.D., Borriello, S.P., & Mahida, Y.R. (2004). Colonic IgA producing cells and macrophages are reduced in recurrent and non-recurrent *Clostridium difficile*-associated diarrhoea. Journal of Clinical Pathology, 57: 973.

18. Gerding et al., 1995.

19. Johnson & Gerding, 1998.

20. Fekety, R. (1997). Guidelines for the diagnosis and management of *Clostridium difficile*-associated diarrhea and colitis. The American Journal of Gastroenterology, 92: 739.

21. Association for Professionals in Infection Control and Epidemiology. (2008). National Prevalence Study of *Clostridium difficile* in U.S. Healthcare Facilities. Washington, D.C.: APIC.

22. Gerding et al., 1995.

23. Dial, S., Delaney, J.A.C., Barkun, A.N., Suissa, S. (2005). Use of Gastric acid–suppressive agents and the risk of community-acquired *Clostridium difficile*–associated disease. Journal of the American Medical Association, 294: 2989.

24. Parente, F., Cucino, C., Gallus, S., Bargiggia, S., Greco, S., Pastore, L., Bianchi Porro, G. (2003). Hospital use of acid-suppresive medications and its fall-out on prescribing in general practice: a 1-month survey. Alimentary Pharmacology and Therapeutics, 17: 1503.

25. Gerding et al., 1995.

26. Bartlett, 2008.

27. Isakow, W., Morrow, L.E., & Kollef, M.H. (2007). Probiotics for pre-

venting and treating nosocomial infections: Review of current evidence and recommendations. Chest, 132: 286.

28. Monaghan, T., Boswell, T., & Mahida, Y. (2008). Recent advances in *Clostridium difficile*-associated disease. Gut, 57: 850.

29. McFarland, L.V., Mulligan, M.E., Kwok, R.Y.Y., & Stamm, W.E. (1989). Nosocomial acquisition of *Clostridium difficile* infection. The New England Journal of Medicine, 320: 204.

30. Halsey, 2008.

31. Gerding et al., 1995.

32. Kelly, Pothoulakis, & LaMont, 1994.

33. Gerding et al., 1995.

34. Halsey, 2008.

35. Nylund, C.M., Goudie, A., Garza, J.M., Fairbrother, G., Cohen, M.B. (2011). *Clostridium difficile* infection in hospitalized children in the United States. Archives of Pediatrics & Adolescent Medicine, 165(5), 451.

36. Rahmani R, et al "Aspirin prevents the development of *C. difficile* associated diarrhea in hospitalized patients" ACG 2010; Abstract 401.

37. Kyne, L., Merry, C., O'Connell, B., Keane, C., & O'Neill, D. (1998). Community-acquired *Clostridium difficile* infection. Journal of Infection, 36: 287.

38. Songer, J.G., Trinh, H.T., Killgore, G.E., Thompson, A.D., McDonald, L.C., Limbago, B.M. (2009). *Clostridium difficile* in retail meat products, USA, 2007. Emerging Infectious Diseases, 15(5): 819.

39. McDonald, L.C., Killgore, G.E., Thompson, A., Owens, Jr., R.C., Kazakova, S.V., Sambol, S.P., Johnson, S., & Gerding, D.N. (2005). An epidemic, toxin gene-variant strain of *Clostridium difficile*. The New England Journal of Medicine, 353: 2433.

40. Warney, M., Pepin, J., Fang, A., Killgore, G., Thompson, A., Brazier, J., Frost, E., & McDonald, L.C. (2005). Toxin production by an emerging straing of *Clostridium difficile* associated with outbreaks of severe disease in North America and Europe. Lancet, 366: 1079.

41. Warney et al., 2005.

Chapter Two
Diagnosing and Treating C. difficile

When to Suspect C. diff

You probably wouldn't have bought this book if you didn't already know that you (or your loved one) have C. diff, but for the sake of thoroughness, we want to talk about how doctors diagnose C. diff.

First and foremost, your doctor will suspect C. diff if you've had antibiotics within the last few months, and have watery, mucousy, or bloody diarrhea three or more times a day that lasts for more than a few days. Recall from Chapter One that some diarrhea is common after antibiotics, and isn't necessarily an indicator of C. diff. However, run-of-the-mill antibiotic-associated diarrhea is relatively mild and short-lived, typically lasting no more than a few days. If your diarrhea lasts longer than this, or worsens over time, a check for C. diff is in order. We should also mention that there are *lots* of other causes of diarrhea, including viruses, food poisoning, irritable bowel syndrome, ulcerative colitis, and many others. If you have diarrhea but haven't had antibiotics recently, it's likely your doctor will exhaust these other possibilities before exploring the C. diff diagnosis.

Additionally, while increasing age (over 65 years old) and antibiotic use remain the first and strongest risks factor for C. diff infection, doctors have now identified other contributing risk factors that may tip them off to a C. diff infection. These include: being female, having a weakened immune system or inflammatory bowel disease, exposure to immunosuppressive agents, gastrointestinal surgery, stool softeners, gastrointestinal stimulants, antiperistaltic drugs, proton-pump inhibitors (and other medications that reduce stomach acidity), and very, very rarely, enemas[1]. Before you let these other risk factors alarm you, it is important to remember that the risk these factors contribute is comparatively small, and you should never stop taking medicines your doctor has prescribed without consulting with him or her first.

Testing for C. diff

If your doctor does suspect C. diff, she will most likely order a series of tests to confirm her suspicions. In the section below, we talk about the variety of tests your doctor might order, but it's important to remember that she may use all or none of these. C. diff diagnosis can be as much art as science, and different doctors will have different preferences for testing.

Stool Tests

The most commonly used diagnostic tools for detecting C. diff are the many and varied stool tests. The various tests are quite complex and

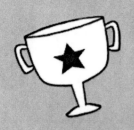

In October 2005 I ate some pumpkin seeds from an open bin in my local supermarket. A few hours later, I started having diarrhea every 15 minutes or so. After 24 hours it turned to bright red blood every 15 minutes.

It took over a month (a horrible, trying month) for the doctors to diagnose my C. diff. The gastroenterologist who finally diagnosed it first prescribed Flagyl, which I took for ten days. The diarrhea stopped. Three days after finishing the Flagyl, I relapsed.

This time I took vancomycin for three weeks, but relapsed again. That was a horrible relapse, and they made me wait three days for a stool test result before giving me any more meds. I had bloody diarrhea every 10 - 20 minutes night and day, with fever, nausea, and misery. I lost seven pounds in those three days. The test finally came back positive and I was put on more Vanco.

My gastroenterologist quit on me after saying that I was an "exceptional case." Then I found an infectious diseases doctor. She was much more helpful. I brought her the "pulsing" regimen that I had found on the C. diff support site, plus a reference to a medical paper favorably comparing pulsing with other treatment methods. That is what finally worked for me, after eight months of C. diff. Without the C. diff Web site, I would never have known about it.

The reason that I volunteer on the C. diff site is that without it, who knows where I would be. It was so encouraging to know that I was not alone, that others had beaten this, that I could beat it too, that there was hope! I learned about probiotics, about diet, about post-C. diff problems and so much more. Mostly I learned that I could have my life back!

Kay E., El Cerrito, CA

have absurdly long names like "tissue culture cytotoxicity assay," so we won't go into the technical details of each here. If you're interested in the specifics of the tests, they are discussed in many of the articles cited for this chapter[2]. While these tests all work in different ways, each uses some method to detect the presence of C. diff toxins in stool.

The various stool tests all differ in terms of how accurately they diagnosis C. diff. None of them is perfectly accurate. Some have a high false positive rate, meaning they often deliver a positive diagnosis of C. diff when none is really there. Some have a high false negative rate, meaning they often fail to indicate C. diff when that is really the cause of someone's illness. For example, the Enzymeimmunoassay test (EIA) will catch about 76-87% of the true C. diff infections. That means that 13-24% of the time, this test fails to identify the presence of C. diff

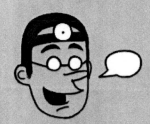

Sensitivity and Specificity: When doctors talk about diagnostic tests, they use two terms to describe the accuracy of the test. "Sensitivity" describes how well the test diagnoses the presence of disease. A doctor could trust a highly "sensitive" test to tell her who had a certain disease. "Specificity" describes how well a test diagnoses the absence of disease. A doctor could trust a highly "specific" test to tell him who didn't have a certain disease. The ideal test would be both very sensitive and very specific. Such a test could be trusted to tell us both who had the disease and who didn't. Unfortunately, there is no such thing as a perfect test. Sometimes the test will tell us someone has a disease, when they really don't, and vice versa. These terms are closely related to a test's false negative and false positive rate.

Test	Sensitivity (%)	Specificity (%)	Processing Time
Stool Culture	>90	80-90	2-4 days
Cytotoxin Assay (only diagnoses toxin B)	75-85	>97	2-3 days
Enzyme Immunoassay (for toxins A & B)	76-87	95	hours to days
Polymerase Chain Reaction (PCR; for toxins A & B)	>90	>97	hours

Table 2.1: Sensitivities and specificities for the most commonly used C. diff diagnostic tests. Remember that sensitivity describes the percentage of patients with C. diff infections that the test will correctly identify as infected, while specificity describes the percentage of C. diff patients without an infection that the test correctly diagnoses as infection-free. As of the writing of this book, the most commonly used test is the cytotoxin assay, but this is likely to rapidly change with the arrival of faster and more accurate PCR tests now on the market. This table constructed partially from data in Poutanen, S.M., & Simor, A.E. (2004). Clostridium difficile-associated diarrhea in adults. Canadian Medical Association Journal, 171: 51.

in someone who really has it. You should also know that until recently, the test with the lowest combined false-positive and false-negative rates (the stool culture, in which C. diff bacteria are grown from a stool sample) had the longest turn around time, up to 96 hours. That means that if your doctor likes to use that test, you're going to be waiting up to a week for your C. diff results.

Until very recently, the most commonly used test was the EIA, and doctors often ordered a series of EIAs for you to do over two to three days. That way, they were able to make sure that the tests done on different days agreed and get the most reliable diagnosis. New, state-of-the-art PCR tests (Polymerase Chain Reaction, a test that looks for the DNA of C. diff toxin-producing genes in your stool) have become the new standard for C. diff detection; they are quick (same day results), accurate and no more difficult to do than any other stool test.

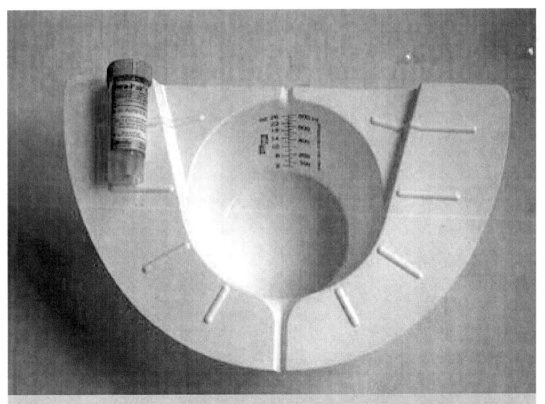

Figure 2.1: A stool collection "hat" and C. diff stool sample vial. The hat is placed over the toilet seat, and used during defecation. A small spoon integrated into the lid of the vial is used to add stool to the fixative fluid in the vial. (photo credit: R. Rizk)

Stool tests are relatively easy to do for the patient, unless they are so ill that even trips to the bathroom are challenging. If you are considered a possible C. diff sufferer, you will be asked to either collect a relatively large amount of stool in a cup-sized container, or to collect a tiny bit of stool in a vial of preservative fluid. Typically, a stool collection "hat" that fits over the toilet seat is provided to aid in collection (see Figure 2.1). The hat is particularly useful if you are having active diarrhea. After collection, both types of samples require quick processing as C. diff toxins break down relatively quickly in the environment. This is one likely explanation for false negative test results. To avoid this, you should store your samples in the fridge and get them to the testing lab as quickly as possible after collection. Processing time varies for the different tests, but you can generally expect results within one to three days.

Blood Tests

There is no blood test that will tell you if you have or don't have C. diff. However, your doctor may order blood tests to see if you have 1) a high white blood cell count, indicating infection, and/or 2) specific blood chemicals called "inflammatory factors," indicating tissue inflammation in your intestines. While neither of these tests will tell your doctor if you have C. diff, they will tell him how sick you are, regardless of what is making you sick. Because your doctor may treat mild C. diff differently than severe C. diff, this is useful information.

Imaging

There are a variety of ways for a doctor to get a picture of your guts, including X-ray, CAT scan, and MRI. Some will show changes in the gut

Testing for cure: The unreliability of these tests, paired with the likelihood that a C. diff sufferer will still carry around the bug for some time after "recovering," is another reason doctors don't like to "test for cure." Even without the presence of C. diff symptoms, there's a good chance a recovering patient will test positive for C. diff, so doctors prefer to wait to retest after treatment unless C. diff symptoms reappear. This can be complicated by the fact that recovery from C. diff takes a long time, and may involve symptoms that appear to be C. diff-like as your gut is healing. More on that fun game in Chapter Four!

that might be caused by C. diff, but not reliably, so using imaging for diagnosis of C. diff is uncommon, and likely to be cross-checked with some of the other tests mentioned in this chapter. Imaging is most likely to be used when a patient is very ill and doctors are interested in getting all the information they can quickly get about the patient's condition.

Gastrointestinal Endoscopy

All endoscopy involves viewing a patient's intestines with a camera-equipped flexible tube inserted into the patient's mouth ("upper endoscopy") or anus (which includes "proctoscopy," "sigmoidoscopy," and "colonoscopy"). Endoscopy is the only way to definitively diagnosis pseudomembranous colitis, the visible damage to the intestines caused by C. diff that we talked about in Chapter One. Unfortunately, endoscopy is expensive, invasive, and not as good at diagnosing C. diff as the newer tests that we talked about in the 'Stool Tests' section above (according to one author, it's inaccurate about 50% of the time[3]). The problem is that many patients have C. diff without having easily visible pseudomembranous colitis. On the other hand, endoscopy does allow a doctor to look for a number of different intestinal problems at one time, so it is used by gastroenterologists who are trying to nail down a tricky diagnosis or looking for complicating factors in patients who are having a hard time getting rid of their C. diff. Endoscopy may also be used for diagnosis when a patient is very ill and doctors don't want to wait for a C. diff stool test. As the PCR stool test becomes more popular, endoscopy may fade as a C. diff diagnostic tool, since processing the PCR test only takes a few hours.

No one looks forward to a colonoscopy (or any other endoscopy, for that matter), but it is relatively safe and routine compared to most other "invasive" procedures. The worst part of the procedure for most patients is the preparation, which involves fasting and purging with laxatives the day before. Ironically, for many C. diff patients, this unpleasantness is just business as usual.

Doctors who don't want to wait to do a colonoscopy may opt to do a flexible sigmoidoscopy instead. In this procedure, only the part of the colon closest to the anus is looked at. This procedure can easily be done without preparation in the outpatient setting. However, because C. diff sometimes shows up only in the right colon — the part of the colon farthest from the anus — it can occasionally be missed by a sigmoidoscopy.

C. diff diagnosis is not necessarily complicated. If a doctor suspects C. diff because of the presence of diarrhea and recent antibiotic use, she will very likely order one or more of the stool tests described above. If those tests come back positive for C. diff, she's very likely to begin treatment right away.

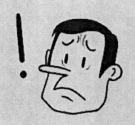 **"My tests are negative, but I know I have C. diff!"** Ask a group of people who've suffered from recurrent C. diff and odds are good that a chunk of them will tell you that at some point during their disease their C. diff tests came back negative, but they were certain they had active disease. This can be a horribly frustrating situation for the patient and doctor alike. There are a number of possible explanations for this situation:

1. They really didn't have C. diff, but instead had post-infectious irritable bowel syndrome, which can mimic C. diff.

2. They were on, or had recently been on, medications that influenced the test. Antibiotics like Flagyl and vancomycin can mask the presence of C. diff up to two weeks after ingestion.

3. The test is wrong. As we mentioned above, no C. diff test is perfect, and it's entirely possible that the test failed to detect the patient's C. diff.

What should you do in this situation? This is a very tough decision, and one that ultimately will be made by you and your doctor. Retesting is a definite possibility, as is waiting a couple more days. If after a few days your symptoms don't improve, some doctors will re-prescribe antibiotics, but others will be very confident about the negative test results and will look for other explanations.

Treating C. diff

Once the dreaded diagnosis of *C. difficile* is made, your doctor has to treat it. The good news is that for most, treatment is simple and quick. The bad news is that for an unlucky minority (15%-30% of patients), their battle with C. diff will not be over as soon. The most important thing for C. diff patients (and their doctors) to remember is that every case of C. diff, and every patient with C. diff, is different. What worked marvelously well for patient A may fail miserably in patient B and lead to the return of the disease soon after the end of treatment. We'll talk more about treating recurrent C. diff in the next chapter.

Cessation of the Inciting Antibiotic

The most important step in treating C. diff is stopping use of the antibiotic that touched off the infection in the first place (assuming antibiotics were involved at all). In 20%-25% of newly onset C. diff, especially if the infection is mild, stopping all antibiotics will lead to a full recovery[4]. Often, the decision to stop antibiotics will be made in the hospital by the attending physician. Because there are usually good reasons a patient is on antibiotics, you should never decide to stop your antibiotics without talking to your doctor. As we mentioned earlier in this chapter, your doctor probably won't stop your antibiotics unless he or she is convinced that you have C. diff, preferably confirmed with a stool test. Of course, because a C. diff infection can blossom up to two or three months after antibiotic use, there may be no antibiotics to stop. In this all too common case, your doctor will almost certainly recommend treating the disease pharmaceutically (more on that in a few pages).

Hydration and Avoidance of Anti-Motility Drugs

Regardless of how C. diff is treated, your doctor will want to make sure your basic bodily functions are supported. As with any diarrhea, the greatest danger of C. diff for most patients is dehydration. Until your doctor has your diarrhea under control, he or she will probably

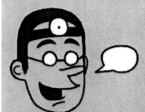

Motility: When doctors use the word "motility," they're most often talking about the speed and comfort by which digesting food (and later waste) is moved through the intestines. Good motility results in pain-free digestion and 1-3 bowel movements a day. When gut motility is impaired and is either too fast or too slow, that can contribute to issues of either constipation or diarrhea, respectively. Anti-motility drugs like Immodium are given during periods of diarrhea to slow the rate of gut motility and give the gut more time to digest the food and remove water content from it.

advise you to "drink plenty of fluids and get plenty of rest." This is good advice, since your body won't fight the infection as well if you're dehydrated and exhausted. As with any persistent diarrhea, small sips of clear liquids between bouts of diarrhea are recommended[5]. If your diarrhea is bad, they might suggest drinking an oral rehydration solution like Pedialyte. And if your diarrhea is so severe that you are dangerously dehydrated, you will likely be advised to get to an emergency room where an IV can be used to get fluids directly into your bloodstream. A word of warning: In cases of severe C. diff, patients can progress from mild dehydration to dangerous dehydration very quickly. If you have any questions about the state of a loved one suffering from severe diarrhea, call your doctor or get to an emergency room as soon as possible.

Unlike your run-of-the-mill diarrhea, C. diff patients should be very careful about taking anti-motility drugs like Lomotil or Immodium[8]. These drugs work by calming down the rapid movements of the intestine that are moving your stool through you too quickly and causing diarrhea. This slowing down is helpful with regular diarrhea, but with C. diff it can keep those C. diff toxins trapped in your intestines, and cause even more damage than normal. However, some doctors will feel comfortable giving anti-motility drugs if the patient is otherwise healthy and treatment is proceeding positively.

Flagyl and vancomycin - The Old Standbys

It is an ironic quirk that antibiotics cause most C. diff infections, and yet antibiotics are used to treat most C. diff infections. For the last 25 years doctors have been successfully treating C. diff with two antibiotics: metronidazole (marketed, and most often referred to, as Flagyl) and vancomycin (sometimes marketed as Vancocin, but most commonly referred to as vancomycin or "vanco").

Is the Treatment Worse Than the disease? Flagyl is a reliable and proven drug for killing off a C. diff infection. Sadly, the side effects of Flagyl are often just as bad as a mild case of C. diff. They include abdominal pain, nausea, loss of appetite, an awful metallic taste in one's mouth, tingling in one's limbs, and even, ironically, diarrhea. Because very long-term use of Flagyl can result in permanent nerve damage, it should not be used for treatment of recurrent C. diff (more on that in Chapter 3). Vancomycin, on the other hand, is a wonderful drug for treating C. diff, as it is not absorbed from the intestine, and thus has no real side effects (with the exception of a common, temporary rash[6]). This non-absorption also makes vancomycin the first treatment of choice for pregnant women with C. diff.

I Don't Want This In Me! It's possible that you have recently tested positive for C. diff without having any symptoms. This outcome is quite common after an infection has been successfully treated, and the numbers of C. diff in your system have been reduced to a harmless level kept in check by your other gut bacteria. You may desperately want this C. diff entirely out you, and might even consider talking your doctor into treating you with more antibiotics to kill them. This would be a bad idea. A commonly-cited study on treating asymptomatic carriers (as this situation is called) found that 9 out of 10 C. diff carriers treated with antibiotics did indeed become culture negative soon after treatment – meaning no C. diff was discovered in their stool – but 70 days later, 4 of those 9 patients were positive again for C. diff, and one even got an active C. diff infection when he or she had had none previously. In the control group, where 9 asymptomatic carriers were simply treated with a placebo, and not antibiotics, only 1 of the 9 tested positive for C. diff at 70 days[7]. Although this was a particularly small study, these findings suggest that given enough time, most patients will kick any residual C. diff out of their system without help from antibiotics.

These drugs are most often taken orally, but can be administered intravenously or via enema in extreme cases.

Flagyl and vancomycin are remarkably similar in efficacy, both in treating mild, active C. diff (each has about a 98%-100% cure rate), and in preventing future recurrences (though there are some minor differences[9]). Recent research has begun to suggest that for severe initial infections of C. diff, or for higher risk patients, vancomycin may actually have the better response rate of the two antibiotics[10]. This, and the fact that patients tend to respond more quickly to vancomycin,[11] is changing initial treatment patterns for high risk patients with severe C. diff. Keep in mind, however, that for less severe C. diff, Flagyl is still the first drug of choice, mainly for cost reasons.

Both Flagyl and vancomycin are most effective when taken for at least 10 days. A typical prescription of Flagyl is 250mg, taken four times a day for 10-14 days. A typical prescription of vancomycin is 125 mg, taken four times a day, also for 10-14 days. There does not appear to be a difference in effectiveness between this dosage of vancomycin and higher doses[12]. It takes about 2-4 days for either drug to kick in and reduce symptoms, and about 2 weeks on average to completely end the diarrhea[13], although some may see results more quickly, and some more slowly.

Where Flagyl and vancomycin really differ is in their cost. As of this writing, Flagyl's pharmacy cost (in the U.S.) is about 40 cents to 70 cents per pill, while vancomycin's is an astonishing $30 per pill (vancomycin is much more difficult to make in pill form than Flagyl). This radical difference in cost, and a fear that C. diff will develop an immunity to vancomycin, leads most doctors to prescribe Flagyl first.

Most patients will wave a permanent goodbye to C. diff after their first round of Flagyl or vancomycin, but about 15%-30% will have a relapse or recurrence of the disease. A second infection of C. diff is called a relapse if it is caused by the same strain that caused the initial infection. It is assumed that relapses are caused by residual C. diff spores coming back to life after the Flagyl or vancomycin treatment is over. A second infection is called a recurrence if it is caused by

Flagyl or metronizadole? Most of the medicines used today have multiple names, and Flagyl is no exception. Flagyl is actually just the "trade name" under which the medicine is marketed in the U.S. and Europe. In other parts of the world, it's called Nidagyl or Megapyl (trade names like these are almost always capitalized). Flagyl's "generic name" is metronizadole. This is the name doctors will quite often use when talking about the drug with each other; that's because the generic name tends to stay the same for a drug regardless of who's making it or where they're selling it. Generic names are generally not capitalized. All drugs have trade names and generic names and it's easy to confuse the two. It gets even crazier when you realize that each drug also has a chemical name. Flagyl's is 2-(2-methyl-5-nitro-1H-imidazol-1-yl)ethanol, but almost nobody worries about those, so you shouldn't either.

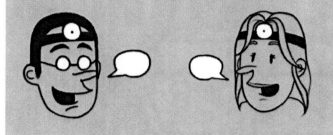

reinfection with a different strain of C. diff. This may sound like a fairly rare occurrence, but more than 50% of repeat C. diff infections are recurrences[14]! An initial relapse or recurrence is no call for panic (for simplicity's sake we'll refer to them both as recurrences from here on out). The vast majority of these are successfully treated with a second round of Flagyl or vancomycin, and are not due to antibiotic resistance (C. diff resistance or resilience to Flagyl does exist, but is quite rare: 6.3% of strains and 3.1% of strains in 2002, respectively[15]). Additionally, should your C. diff come back for a third time or more, doctors have a powerful way to use one of these two antibiotics – generally vancomycin

– called a pulsed-taper. The pulsed-taper is currently the most effective tool for killing recurrent C. diff, and we'll talk more about it in the next chapter.

There are a number of other antibiotics that have been used as frontline treatments for C. diff, notably teicoplanin, bacitracin, and fusicid acid. None of these drugs has proven to be drastically more effective than Flagyl and vancomycin[16], so they are typically not used by doctors. The reality is that Flagyl and vancomycin are so effective for most people that alternative therapies are infrequently needed. However, because doctors differ in terms of treatment philosophies and approaches, we'll finish this section by talking about other drugs and therapies that your doctor might use against your C. diff.

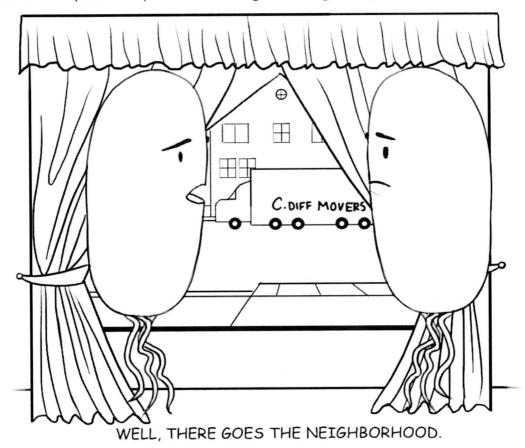

WELL, THERE GOES THE NEIGHBORHOOD.

Probiotics

Just as probiotics can help prevent (
used to treat an active C. diff infecti
"[probiotics] compete for nutrients, s
hibit mucosal adherence, may prod
provide colonization resistance to C.
on probiotics and C. diff has focusec
lardii, and a bacterium called Lactok
research is not entirely conclusive, ar
there does seem to be some benefit
your C. diff treatment regimen. For example, one study found that
vancomycin treatment paired with daily doses of the helpful yeast
Saccharomyces boulardii was 67% more effective in clearing C. diff
than vancomycin treatment alone[19]. Other studies have confirmed the
benefit of probiotics, particularly in reducing the risk of recurrences[20].
This makes sense if we return to our cow metaphor in chapter one.
These friendly probiotic "cows" help to replace the lost "cows" of our
normal gut flora, and crowd out the opportunistic C. diff. There's even
some evidence that probiotics like Saccharomyces boulardii actively
attack C. diff bacteria and C. diff toxins chemically[21] and can prime
the body's immune system to target C. diff toxins[22]!

We must note here that there are some risks to probiotics, particularly for immunosuppressed and debilitated patients. In these cases, it
is possible for the probiotics to cause their own infection in a compromised immune system, creating a new problem for the patient[23]. While
such cases are rare, patients and doctors should weigh the potential
risks and benefits of incorporating probiotics into a C. diff

...en I have C. diff? To our knowledge, no ... the impact of different diets on recovery ... reality is that when your C. diff is active, you ...like eating much at all. A suppressed appetite is ...possible symptoms of C. diff, and there's the problem ...ing tends to result in more diarrhea, which is uncom-...ble. Many C. diff patients are encouraged to stay on the ...RAT diet for a while (bananas, rice, applesauce, and toast). If this makes you feel better, than by all means do so, but many doctors worry about the lack of balanced nutrition in the BRAT diet and would not want you on it for a long period of time. The debate is still on in this particular area.

Believe it or not, a number of studies suggest adding Indian food to your C. diff diet! Curcurmin, a spice found in many Indian curry powders, appears to inhibit C. difficile growth, and has long been used as a general gastric aid in India. We can't recommend this particular home cure just yet; for one thing, this research is quite new and little is known about how curcurmin interacts with other medicines.

The only hard-and-fast rule of eating while active with C. diff is to get plenty of fluids into you. Try frequent small sips  of water, popsicles, oral rehydration fluids like Pedialyte, or broth. While you can go for some time without eating, you absolute can't go without drinking. You should carefully monitor yourself for signs of dehydration (e.g. lack of saliva, dizziness, loss of skin elasticity) and seek medical help if you are dangerously dehydrated.

treatment plan, especially if the patient is immunosuppressed or otherwise severely compromised.

Some experts also recommend using "prebiotics" to boost the growth of beneficial bacteria. Although they sound similar to probiotics, prebiotics aren't bacteria at all. Instead they are indigestible food ingredients (fructo-oligosaccharides being one of the most common) that feed good bacteria[24]. Research on the impact of prebiotics on C. diff is limited, however, and we encourage you to talk to your doctor before including them in your diet.

Sequestrants

Sequestrants include resins like Cholestrymine and powders like activated charcoal that easily bind other chemicals and render them harmless. Sequestrants are given orally to C. diff patients to bind the C. diff toxins in their guts and carry them out of their systems. This is a neat idea, since it is the toxins that do all the damage in a C. diff infection. Clinical studies in which sequestrants were paired with antibiotics have shown promising results[25]. Unfortunately, sequestrants can also bind any medicines in your system (like the antibiotics being used to treat C. diff) and render them inactive as well. So, if your doctor does prescribe a sequestrant, make sure you take it as far from the time you are taking your medicines as you can (e.g., if you are taking your antibiotic at 8 a.m. and noon, take the sequestrant at 10 a.m.).

Surgery and Extreme Medication Delivery

In a very small percent (<3%) of C. diff infections, the patient will present with a condition called "toxic megacolon." In this scary (but rare)

Do I have toxic megacolon!!?? At some point in your C. diff treatment, your diarrhea will stop. At this point, if you are the worrying sort, you may convince yourself that you have toxic megacolon for the sole reason that you had diarrhea for a long time and now you don't. Rest assured that your doctor will recognize the difference between toxic megacolon and "just getting better." For one thing, patients with toxic megacolon will not feel better; they will have severe pain, fever, rapid heartbeat and other symptoms of shock, like pale, clammy skin and trouble staying awake. It is not something you can confuse with improving health. As we've said before, it's very easy to let your fears get the better of you when you have C. diff. Don't let that happen!

situation, the patient's colon has become too poisoned and bloated to work and has essentially stopped most or all functions, including movement of stool through the colon. This lack of stool movement leads to a decrease or even a cessation of diarrhea, which might look like a good sign, but in this case, absolutely isn't. This is an extraordinarily dangerous situation, and about 24%-38% of patients with toxic megacolon will die from it. Doctors sometimes try to treat this condition by introducing high dosage liquid antibiotics to the gut via nasogastric tube or enema[26], but quite often the only lifesaving procedure they can employ is an almost total colectomy — removal of the colon. Even then, the procedure is dangerous, and many do not survive.

C. diff and Inflammatory Bowel Disease

Earlier in this chapter we mentioned that Inflammatory Bowel Disease (IBD) was one of the factors that increased a patient's chances of contracting C. diff. In the USA, between 1998 and 2004, for every 1,000 patient discharges, C. diff was nearly eight times more likely among IBD patients than non-IBD patients [10]. Antibiotics are still the main culprit for the majority (61%) of C. diff infections in IBD patients[27]. IBD also drastically complicates the progression and severity of an active C. diff infection. IBD encompasses two different but closely related conditions: Crohn's disease and ulcerative colitis. Both diseases cause chronic inflammation of the gastrointestinal system and sometimes inflammation outside the gastrointestinal system.

Gastrointestinal inflammation can manifest in many different ways for the IBD patient. Damage to the mucosa can result in ulcerations, scarring and deeper penetration into the adjacent tissue, called an abscess. Both diseases can involve other parts of the body including the spine, joints and eyes. Ulcerative colitis is typically restricted to the colon, whereas Crohn's disease can range from mouth to anus. Crohn's disease tends to be patchy, whereas the inflammation from ulcerative colitis tends to be continuous throughout the affected area. There are numerous other differences that doctors use to distinguish the two, and correctly diagnosing a patient with IBD is important because they are treated differently.

This difference in diagnosis and treatment becomes especially important for the patient with C. diff who has IBD of the colon. Recent evidence has shown higher complication rates for patients with ulcerative colitis (UC) who develop C. diff. Specifically, UC patients need longer hospitalization, are more likely to require colectomy (surgical removal of the colon) and have higher mortality rates than Crohn's disease patients. When we consider the impact of C. diff on IBD, it is important to answer a few important frequently asked questions.

Question: Does C. diff cause IBD ?

Answer: No, C. diff infection alone does not cause IBD. The causes of IBD are not well understood, but most IBD investigators feel that there is an interaction among three important elements:

1. The patient's genetic predisposition: We know that patients who have a first degree relative with IBD (mother, father, siblings and children) have a much higher risk of developing IBD.

2. The patient's history of environmental exposure: Gor some unexplained reason, people living in more developed countries have a higher risk of IBD then people who live in developing countries. It's not clear why this might be, but some researchers think it may be linked to changes in the intestinal flora of citizens of developed countries.

3. The patient's immune system: Differences in an individual's immune response to infection, diet, stress and unknown factors seem to influence the occurrence of IBD. Patients with some types of autoimmune diseases are more likely to develop IBD.

Let's look at an example of where a patient could be confused into believing that C. diff caused her IBD: 23-year-old Amanda was initially diagnosed with severe Irritable Bowel Syndrome after several months of diarrhea and urgency to go to the bathroom. During a second round of testing, her doctors found C. diff even though she hadn't

64

been on antibiotics anytime in the recent past. Despite successful eradication of C. diff, she continued to have bouts of diarrhea through the day and sometimes at night. The nighttime diarrhea is one clue that her ongoing symptoms cannot simply be attributed to "Irritable Bowel Syndrome worse after C. diff."

As weeks go by, she begins to have even more nighttime diarrhea. She loses weight and cannot complete a day of work in the office. Her physician suggests a third round of testing, including blood work and a colonoscopy, and that is when she is finally diagnosed with ulcerative colitis. In Amanda's case, the best explanation for why C. diff was diagnosed before IBD is straightforward. Most likely, the IBD was there all along from the very beginning of her illness, and then she

GI? ID? PCP? Doctors and the folks who work with them use a lot of different acronyms to make talking to each other a little bit easier. Your PCP is your Primary Care Provider, quite often a specialist in family or internal medicine who handles your day-to-day health complaints and identifies more serious issues. Your C. diff journey is likely to begin (and hopefully end) with your PCP. Patients with more persistent or more worrisome cases of C. diff are likely to be sent to a GI or gastroenterologist, or an ID, an infectious disease specialist. Gastroenterologists study disorders of the digestive system. They may see patients with chronic acid reflux, liver disease, gall bladder stones, or worries

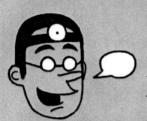

about colon cancer all in the same day. They also see lots of patients with C. diff. Infectious Disease specialists specialize in the treatment of diseases caused by infectious agents; this would include bacterial diseases like C. diff and Legionnaire's Disease, but could also include viral diseases or parasitic infections.

acquired C. diff which made her UC even more severe. Amanda must now start the journey of treating her UC and preventing any recurrent C. diff.

Question: Can C. diff dramatically worsen IBD?

Answer: Most IBD patients who receive antibiotic treatment do respond well and are cured of C. diff. For a significant minority, however, C. diff infection can dramatically worsen the course of IBD, especially when the IBD involves the colon. Some patients' IBD condition may worsen so much that they need to have their colon surgically removed (colectomy) to control or eliminate the disease.

Let's consider another case that may help illustrate this situation: Max is a 30-year-old roofer who has had well-controlled UC for five years. Max needed good control because he can't get to a bathroom quickly when working on top of a roof! During his fifth year of treatment (which included medications to wean his immune system off steroids), he developed a bad flare-up of his UC.

This flare-up occurred a few weeks after treatment for sinusitis with antibiotics. Fortunately, his doctors recognized that his flare-up might be due to C. diff. They tested early for the beastly bug (he tested positive) and treated him first with metronidazole. The metronidazole didn't eliminate the C. diff, so they treated him a second time with vancomycin. The vanco worked, but although the bug was gone, Max was not back to normal.

In fact, Max did not respond well enough to go back to work, and his diarrhea and bleeding worsened over three months. He needed to go back on steroids and even more medications to 'help his immune system' overcome the UC. He was finally admitted to a hospital with recurrent dehydration. After many failed attempts to control his disease, Max ultimately needed to have a colectomy to eliminate the UC so that he could go back to work on the rooftops.

Max has a story that is rare, but sadly not as rare as we'd like it to be. Investigators in Milwaukee found that even with proper treatment, 25% of IBD patients required colectomies after C. diff treatment[28]. This occurs much more frequently in UC than in Crohn's disease of the colon. These investigators suggested early treatment for C. diff with vancomycin instead of metrondiazole as one way to possibly reduce the risk of colectomy (but that theory has still not been proved in a rigorously designed trial). Similarly, a British study found that IBD patients who contracted C. diff were more than twice as likely to need a colectomy than other C. diff sufferers[29]. Very early in the C. diff infection in an IBD patient, we can not reliably predict who will be able to avoid colectomy and who will succumb to colectomy. Some clues that suggest the need for colectomy will be higher include age (older than 65 years) and patients who need to be treated in the intensive care unit[30]. These are rough guides however, and we still need to watch carefully every patient

Why the disagreement? You may be wondering why we report a range as large as 15%-30% for recurrence rates. That's because, like many things in science and medicine, different studies report different numbers. Instead of giving you an average of these studies, we've chosen to report the range. Some studies report recurrence rates as low as 15%, while others report rates as high as 30%.

who has IBD of the colon and develops a C. diff infection.

In addition to higher rates of colectomy, some patients with C. diff and IBD who are admitted to the hospital do not survive due to complications. This sad outcome occurs more often in patients with IBD and C. diff compared with C. diff alone. This, fortunately, is an uncommon event, reported in only 3%-4% of such patients during a 2003 study period[31]. And we hope the number will decline further as awareness about treatment increases.

If you are reading this section and have IBD of the colon, especially if you have UC, it is important to be reassured and remember that the surgical techniques for colectomy and restoring bowel continuity are very advanced and successful for the UC patient who is the right candidate. Furthermore, we must first remind everyone with IBD who might be reading this that most patients with IBD make it through a C. diff infection by responding to antibiotics without any need for colectomy.

Recurrence

As we mentioned earlier, most patients with C. diff will be cured in one or two doses of antibiotics. Unfortunately, a sizable minority (15%-30% of patients) will suffer from repeated recurrences of C. diff infection. As we discussed above, the antibiotic cure for C. diff also leaves the gut empty of protective bacteria and susceptible to another bout of the disease as residual spores sprout in the intestines. This vicious cycle can go on for some time. Patients who suffer one relapse are 65% more likely to have another one[32]. In Chapter Three, we discuss the trials of recurrent C. diff, and look at ways to treat the disease.

Notes – Chapter Two

1.   Halsey, J. (2008). Current and future treatment modalities for *Clostridium difficile*-associated disease. American Journal of Health-System Pharmacy, 65: 705.

2.   Bartlett, J.G. (2008). Historical perspectives on studies of *Clostridium difficile* and *C. difficile* infection. Clinical Infectious Diseases, 46: S4., and Poutanen, S.M., & Simor, A.E. (2004). *Clostridium difficile*-associated diarrhea in adults. Canadian Medical Association Journal, 171: 51.

3.   Gerding, D.N, Johnson, S., Peterson, L.R., Mulligan, M.E., & Silva, Jr., J. (1995). *Clostridium difficile*-associated diarrhea and colitis. Infection Control and Hospital Epidemiology, 16: 459.

4.   Gerding et al., 1995.

5.   Dorner, B. (2007). Nutrition therapy for *C. difficile* diarrhea. Downloaded from assistedlivingconsult.com, May 2011.

6.   McFarland, L.V. (2005). Alternative treatments for *Clostridium difficile* disease: What really works? Journal of Medical Microbiology, 54: 101.

7.   Gerding et al., 1995.

8.   McFarland, 2005.

9.   Poutanen and Simor, 2004.

10.   Zar, F.A., Bakkanagari, S.R., Moorthi, K.M.L.S.T., & Davis, M.B. (2007). A comparison of vancomycin and metronidazole for the treatment of *Clostridium difficile*-associated diarrhea, stratified by disease severity. Clinical Infectious Diseases, 45: 302.

11.   Halsey, 2008.

12.   Halsey, 2008.

13.   McFarland, 2005.

14.   McFarland, 2005.

15.   Halsey, 2008.

16.   Halsey, 2008.

17.   Segarra-Newnham, M. (2007). Probiotics for *Clostridium difficile*–Associated Diarrhea: Focus on Lactobacillus rhamnosus GG

and *Saccharomyces boulardii*. The Annals of Pharmacotherapy, 41: 1212.

18. Dendukuri, N., Costa, V., McGregor, M., & Brophy, J.M. (2005). Probiotic therapy for the prevention and treatment of *Clostridium dfficile*-associated diarrhea: A systematic review. Canadian Medical Association Journal, 173(2): 167.

19. Tonna, I., & Welsby, P.D. (2005). Pathogenesis and treatment of *Clostridium difficile* infection. Postgraduate Medical Journal, 81: 367.

20. Segarra-Newnham, 2007.

21. Castagliuolo, I., Riegler, M.F., Valenick, L., LaMont, J.T., & Pothoulakis, C. (1999). *Saccharomyces boulardii* protease inhibits the effects of *Clostridium difficile* toxins A and B in human colonic mucosa. Infection and Immunity, 67(1): 302.

22. Qamar, A., Aboudola, S., Warny, M., Michetti, P., Pothoulakis, C., LaMont, J.T., & Kelly, C.P. (2001). *Saccharomyces boulardii* intestinal immunoglobulin A immune response to *Clostridium difficile* toxin A in mice. Infection and Immunity, 69(4): 2762.

23. Segarra-Newnham, 2007.

24. Dorner, 2007.

25. Halsey, 2008.

26. Gerding et al., 2995

27. Issa, M., Vijayapal, A., Graham, M.B., Beaulieu, D.B., Otterson, M.F., Lundeen, S., Skaros, S., Weber, L.R., Komorowski, R.A., Knox, J.F., Emmons, J., Bajaj, J.S., & Binion, D.G. (2007). Impact of *Clostridium difficile* on inflammatory bowel disease. Clinical Gastroenterology and Hepatology, 5(3): 345.

28. Ananthakrishnan, A.N., McGinley, E.L., & Binion, D.G. (2007). Excess hospitalization burden associated with *Clostridium difficile* in patients with inflammatory bowel disease. Gut, 57: 150.

29. Jen, M-H., Saxena, S., Bottle, A., Aylin, P., & Pollok, R.C.G. (2011). Increased health burden associated with *Clostridium difficile* diarrhoea in patients with inflammatory bowel disease. Alimentary Pharmacology & Therapeutics, 33(12): 1322.

30. Ananthakrishnan et al., 2007.

31. Jen et al. 2011.

32. Halsey, 2008.

Chapter Three
Recurrent C. difficile

The summer of 2008 was a tough one for Chris, one of the authors of this book. His wife, Victoria, had been suffering from repeated breast infections while trying to nurse their new baby, Madeleine. These painful, scary lumps had necessitated multiple rounds of antibiotics to clear. When they thought things were getting better, Chris' wife came down with a case of persistent, painful diarrhea that was finally diagnosed after three weeks as *C. difficile*. Both Chris and Victoria were terrified by the new and unknown diagnosis. They were even more terrified by their doctor's mysterious warnings to cancel their vacation and stay near a major hospital.

On the advice of another doctor, they didn't cancel their vacation, and they were thrilled when the Flagyl that Victoria had been prescribed cleared up the infection within a day. She felt better than she'd felt in weeks. They returned from their weeklong vacation to a healthy and happy home. Sadly, all of that was quickly shattered.

A few days after Victoria's 10-day run of Flagyl, she and Chris enjoyed a pizza from a local pizza house. The next day, they both had symptoms of food poisoning. Unfortunately, their food poisoning didn't clear up as they expected. Instead, their diarrhea got worse and they began to suspect that Victoria had relapsed into another C. diff infection, and that this time, Chris had joined her as he too became ill. Stool tests confirmed their worst fears: They both had C. diff. They would never know if the pizza had kicked off this new round of sickness, or if they were doomed to C. diff for some other reason. They did know that Chris had taken antibiotics recently for a sinus infection, and that Victoria, of course, had just finished a round of Flagyl. Antibiotics had struck again, and now two people had C. diff.

While Victoria would recover from C. diff after one more round of Flagyl, Chris wouldn't be so lucky. He would go on to have five recurrences of C. diff lasting from July 2009 to February 2010. Sadly, he's not alone; between 15% and 30% of C. diff sufferers will have one or more recurrences, and those who have one recurrence are more likely to have another[1]; in rare (very rare) cases, patients have been known to have ten or more recurrences. If you're reading this book, then it's very likely that you or a loved one is suffering from recurrent C. diff. By reading Chapters One and Two, you should have a good idea of how C. diff happens, and how it is diagnosed and treated in its simplest form. In this chapter, we'll talk about treatments for recurrent C. diff, both conventional and alternative, and the research behind their efficacy.

Could my dog/cat/cockatoo be giving me C. diff? Patients with recurrent C. diff start to see C. diff everywhere. Doorknobs, faucets, linens; everything becomes suspect as a source of re-contamination. An obvious question for the C. diff pet owner is "Could my pet be carrying C. diff and producing spores that then reinfect me?" The answer, unfortunately, is "maybe." C. diff has been found as a relatively common gut bacterium of dogs, cats, livestock like cows, pigs, and horses, and even some birds[2]. Like humans, animals are more likely to carry C. diff after they've been given antibiotics. The samples collected from these various animals were sometimes of the toxin-producing variety and sometimes not. Of the toxic C. diff collected, a large percentage of it was known to be capable of producing disease in humans. However, like humans, C. diff carriage in animals without symptoms of C. diff disease tended to be short-lived. So, should

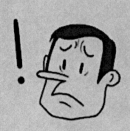 you get rid of your seemingly healthy pet if you have recurrent C. diff? Probably not. Should you get your animal checked out by the vet if they have diarrhea at the same you're suffering from C. diff? Definitely so. Should you be extra careful with your pet's stool when you're trying to get over recurrent C. diff? Probably.

Before we get into the ins and outs of treating recurrent C. diff, let's start on a positive note by reiterating that the majority of C. diff sufferers (upwards of 80% by some estimates) will have their infection cleared by one or two doses of a first-line antibiotic like Flagyl. For those who do have one or more recurrences, there is further good news in that recurrences of C. diff are generally no worse than the initial episode[3], so for most patients, the disease will not get worse each time you have it. In fact, each round may seem easier as you and your doctor become quicker and more effective at diagnosing and treating the disease. Additionally, we can be encouraged by the fact that the vast majority of C. diff recurrences are not due to antibiotic resistance in the bacterium, but are instead due to those pesky spores hanging out until the medicine is gone and then sprouting again[4].

How do I Know it's a Recurrence?

A C. diff infection, even a minor one, can cause damage to the large intestine that may take days, weeks or even months to heal. Most C. diff patients will have some residual disturbance in their stool pattern for some time after they've beaten C. diff. Even if your gut heals quickly, it's important to remember that the antibiotics that killed your C. diff also killed a lot of your other gut bacteria. Until your gut flora recovers, things may be a little iffy, and a small percentage of C. diff patients will suffer from Irritable Bowel Syndrome (also known as IBS; more on this in Chapter Four) for some time after C. diff. This iffy-ness can make diagnosing a C. diff recurrence very tricky; what looks a lot like C. diff may not be. So if you have an episode of diarrhea a short time after getting over a C. diff infection, don't panic. Yes, it may be C. diff returning, but it's equally likely, if not more so, that it's not. Taking more antibiotics is the right decision if it is C. diff, but absolutely

PI-IBS: One term your doctor may bandy about after you've been treated for C. diff is Post-infectious Irritable Bowel Syndrome, or PI-IBS. This simply refers to the dysfunction of the intestines that commonly follows gut infections. We'll talk more about this phenomenon in the next chapter, but for now, rest assured that it is a common occurrence, and often temporary.

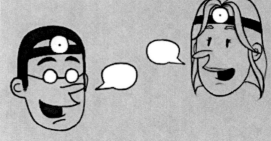

the wrong one if it is not. Remember, each round of antibiotics carries with it a chance of C. diff recurrence. So what can you do?

Be patient

If your diarrhea is not severe, and there is no blood, consider waiting to treat it. On the C. diff forums at www.cdiffsupport.com, patients live by the "Three Day Rule": wait three days to see if your diarrhea improves on its own. Severe IBS episodes can easily last three days and can seem very much like C. diff while they are occurring. However, IBS episodes typically will improve with time, while C. diff typically will not. We should make special note here: Bloody diarrhea is NOT a symptom of IBS and should be assessed by your doctor immediately. Bright red drops of blood when you wipe could be simply hemorrhoids, but blood in the diarrhea requires assessment by your physician.

Call your doctor

Let your doctor know what symptoms you're having and wait to hear from him or her before doing anything else.

Look at the calendar

Most recurrences of C. diff occur three or four days after antibiotic treatment ends, and 97% of recurrences occur within four weeks[5]. If it's been more than a month since your C. diff infection resolved, chances are good your new diarrhea isn't C. diff.

Get a C. diff test

Many patients with recurrent C. diff are certain they can tell when they are having a recurrence and when they are not. They will often arrange with their doctors to have extra antibiotics on hand so that they can begin treatment the moment a recurrence happens. While this rapid-fire approach is understandable, there is always the risk that a patient is wrong, and that they are prolonging their recovery by treating a disease that isn't really there. At the very least, we advise testing stools for C. diff before antibiotics are resumed, as the antibiotics themselves can lead to false positives or false negatives on a number of the older C. diff assays (it's unclear if antibiotics will have the same effect on the new PCR tests).

Stay positive and don't panic

Even if this is another recurrence, you WILL eventually get rid of this bug. Essentially everyone eventually does. It is very easy to let C. diff run you down both physically and emotionally, but it is NOT a permanent state.

Why Do I Have This Again?

Getting C. diff once is painful, scary and debilitating. Getting C. diff multiple times is devastating. It also goes against everything we've learned about infectious diseases as patients. For most of us in developed countries, we get an infection, we go to the doctor, we get an antibiotic, and a few days later we're healthy again. C. diff doesn't obey those rules of illness that we've learned to count on and live by. Doctors are just as frustrated by multiply-recurrent C. diff as patients are. They too are used to modern medicines working well and hate this disease just as much as their patients do.

If you've had C. diff once and have suffered a second (or third, or fourth!) recurrence, you are undoubtedly sad, angry and wondering why this is happening to you. So let's start by looking at why this is happening, and what we can do to stop it. In Chapter Four, we'll tackle those bigger emotional issues that go along with C. diff.

The answer to "Why do I have C. diff again?" is very similar to the answer to that first question we asked back in Chapter One, "Why did I get C. diff in the first place?" Most likely, you got C. diff the first time around due to exposure to antibiotics, and then subsequent exposure to C. diff (as we've mentioned, it's possible to get C. diff without exposure to antibiotics, but it's much rarer). Now,

Resistant? Probably not. One thing we are sure of is that recurrent C. diff is almost never due to resistance to the antibiotics used to treat it. While there are a number of C. diff strains out there that are resistant to some common antibiotics, very few C. diff strains are currently resistant to Flagyl[6], and none that we know of are resistant to vancomycin[7].

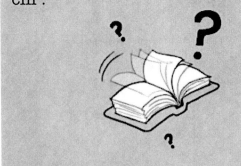

ironically, the antibiotics that your doctor gave you to treat that initial bout of C. diff have left your gut just as empty of beneficial bacteria as it was before.

Essentially, every time doctors treat C. diff with antibiotics, they are hoping that they knock the C. diff back enough for your regular gut flora to return before the C. diff does. All it takes is a few leftover C. diff spores in your gut, or exposure to C. diff spores in the environment, and bam! You're right back where you started. You may think that this comes down to luck of the draw, and to some degree it does, but as

I was a 27-year-old wife and mom of two boys when C. diff first struck. My husband was deployed to Iraq, and I had just decided to return to work after my youngest, Bryton, turned five months old. Bryton immediately picked up a virus in daycare, and soon I had caught it as well. I was put on Biaxin at the time for possible bronchitis, and he was put on amoxicillin for an ear infection.

Immediately, I noticed things weren't right and called the doctor. the doctor assured me all was fine and to continue taking the antibiotic. That was Thursday. By Sunday night, I was in the E.R., sick as I had ever been. The doctor immediately suspected C. diff and started treatment while waiting for a stool test. It was positive. I had no idea what C. diff was or what precautions to take and shortly thereafter, Bryton showed the same symptoms. A positive test revealed that I had passed it to him. We were both put on Metronidazole and Florastor, a yeast probiotic. He had a horrible time taking the Metronidazole because the flavor made him gag, but we both made it through the course of treatment.

I had to adjust to our new "normal." Things definitely were not what they were pre-C. diff. We were blessed enough to both make it a decent amount of time with no relapse. On the 70th day Bryton contracted a stomach virus and another positive test showed C. diff had returned. This time he could not keep the Metronidazole down so we tried Vanco in liquid form. He took to it very well. After a six-week taper and Florastor, he beat C. diff for the second time. He is now almost three years old and is a healthy, happy boy.

Since this episode, we haven't been faced with the dilemma of needing to give him more antibiotics, but we will face that bump in the road when we get to it. I have had two C. diff relapses, each a year apart,

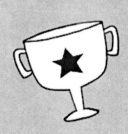

but I've beat C. diff in the past and I'm confident I will beat it again. I do not let it decide who I am, or how much I will live and enjoy my life. I live my life to the fullest despite C. diff. Only you can decide the power C. diff will have in your life.

Amanda L., Bondurant, IA

Reinfection versus relapse: Doctors use a couple of different words when talking about recurrent C. diff. When someone gets another C. diff infection due to leftover spores in their guts hatching and becoming a nuisance again, this is called a "relapse." When someone gets a second (or third, or fourth...) C. diff infection, and it's from a 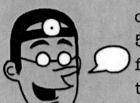 new strain of C. diff in the environment, this is called a "reinfection." Believe it or not, about 50% of all recurrences of C. diff are from a different strain than the one that initially infected the patient[8]. For purposes of simplicity, we'll use the single term "recurrence" for all of these different situations.

we mentioned in Chapter One, there is one last piece of the puzzle here, and that is you.

There is a lot of research coming to light that suggests that a key arbiter in the cycle of C. diff infection is how well your body recognizes and attacks C. diff. For example, in one study[9], researchers found that individuals who mounted a strong immune response to C. diff were less likely to show symptoms from an infection and less likely to have recurrent infections. In this study, the researchers used the number of infection-fighting cells in gut samples from different patients as their measure of an immune response. Those who showed the fewest symptoms had the highest numbers of infection-fighting cells present in the walls of their large intestines. Other studies of the immune response to C. diff have supported this basic conclusion[10].

The sad reality is that if you've gotten C. diff more than once or twice, the ultimate culprit is most likely your own body. Chris, one of the authors of this book, an otherwise healthy man in his 30s, had C. diff five times. He is likely one of those unfortunates who does not mount an effective immune response to C. diff. Before you feel too sorry for him, though, you should know that he got over his infections, and as of the publication of this book, has been C. diff-free for over two years. He has even taken antibiotics for another infection without contracting C. diff! In the next section of this chapter, we'll talk about what you and your doctor can do in the short term to stop the cycle of recurrence. In the long term, you'll want to turn to Chapter Five and learn about the exciting work going on in the realm of C. diff vaccines. This work holds our real possibilities for making everyone resistant to C. diff, regardless of what their own immune response is like.

First-line Treatments for Recurrent C. diff

Let's presume that your stool has been tested, and your doctor believes you're having your first (or second, or third...) C. diff infection; what do you do now? As we mentioned in Chapter Two, your doctor will very likely choose to treat a first recurrence of C. diff with the same medication she used to treat the first occurrence – most often this will be another 10-14 day run of Flagyl or vancomycin. This is the recommended approach, since, as we mentioned before, failures in treating C. diff are almost never due to resistance to the antibiotic, and in fact, what didn't work the first time often *does* work the second time. It's in those cases where two treatments of Flagyl or vancomycin fail that your doctor will need to think more creatively about how to treat you.

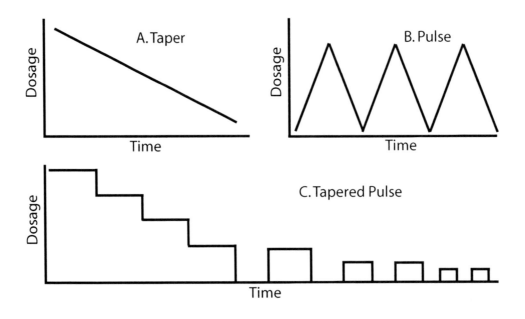

Figure 3.1: A graphical representation of different treatment protocols aimed at elimination recurrent C. diff. A) Tapered protocols steadily drop the dosage of antibiotic taken each day until treatment ends. B) Pulsed protocols take time off between high doses of antibiotic, repeating "antibiotic-on" and "antibiotic-off" days over the course of treatment. C) Tapered-pulsed protocols drop the dosage of antibiotic over time, and then pulse low levels of antibiotic for a set period. The tapered-pulse protocol is currently favored for treatment of recurrent C. diff.

So let's assume, sadly, that your C. diff has returned for a third visit (a clear possibility if you thought enough of your C. diff to buy this book). What will your doctor do? Just 10 years ago, the answer to this question could have been almost anything. There were not well-established guidelines for handling recurrent C. diff, and doctors were trying a variety of creative approaches to treating the disease. Since then, things have improved quite a bit, and gastroenterologists and infectious disease specialists have tracked which treatments work best in permanently eliminating recurrent C. diff. So which treatment works best? The answer for most patients is what doctors call a "tapered-pulsed dose" of an antibiotic which is active against C. diff.

Pulsing and Tapering

Pulsing and tapering are two strategies that have been tried for a while to combat recurrent C. diff. Pulsing refers to a strategy where antibiotics are given in high doses every few days, with no antibiotics taken in between. The idea is to use a high dose of antibiotics to kill the active C. diff bacteria in the patient's gut, and then to trick the remaining C. diff spores into "hatching" by stopping all antibiotics. When the antibiotics are stopped, the C. diff spores think the coast is clear and hatch into active bacteria. Then BAM! the doctor hits them with another high dose of antibiotics. This process is repeated until all the spores have been tricked into hatching and are killed off.

Tapering relies on a similar strategy, but when tapering, the doctor slowly weans the patient off antibiotics over a period of days or weeks. As the antibiotic levels in the gut drop, the C. diff spores are tricked into hatching, but there's still just enough antibiotic being administered to kill them. Tapering and pulsing have both been associated with significantly lower recurrence rates than "traditional" treatment protocols[12].

As you might already have guessed, a "tapered-pulse" combines the two strategies of pulsing and tapering, delivering high doses of antibiotics at first, but then slowly lowering the dosage and eventually pulsing the dosage. While there are probably an infinite number of tapering-pulsing formulas that will work to kill recurrent C. diff, the formula most commonly advocated in the medical literature (and one with even lower recurrence rates than pulsing and tapering alone) looks like this[13]:

- *125 mg vancomycin taken four times daily for 14 days, then*

- *125 mg vancomycin taken twice daily for seven days, then*

- *125 mg vancomycin taken once daily for seven days, then*

- *125 mg vancomycin taken once every two days for eight days (four doses), then*

- *125 mg vancomycin taken once every three days for 15 days (five doses).*

You'll notice that the first fourteen days of the tapered-pulse look pretty much like the usual treatment for first- and second-time C. diff.

Can't we just start with that? If tapered-pulses work so well, why not start out with them? You may be wondering why the tapered-pulse isn't the first treatment of choice for doctors if it works so well. Without going into the specifics of artificial selection, suffice it to say that tapered-pulsing does increase the chances of developing antibiotic-resistance in the patient's particular strain of C. diff[11]; the same logic is behind your doctor's admonishment to finish your whole antibiotic prescription and not stop half-way through. Because standard treatment with Flagyl or vancomycin is generally quite effective, and much safer from an antibiotic-resistance point-of-view, doctors are hesitant to use tapered-pulsing unless they have to.

The dosing formula deviates from there, and it's those five weeks of tapering and pulsing that trick those pesky C. diff spores to hatch and then kill them.

Because this dosing method works so well, most doctors consider it the weapon of choice against recurrent C. diff. Should your C. diff recur a third time, your doctor will probably 1) be fairly surprised, since this is rare, and 2) suggest that the tapered-pulse be repeated,

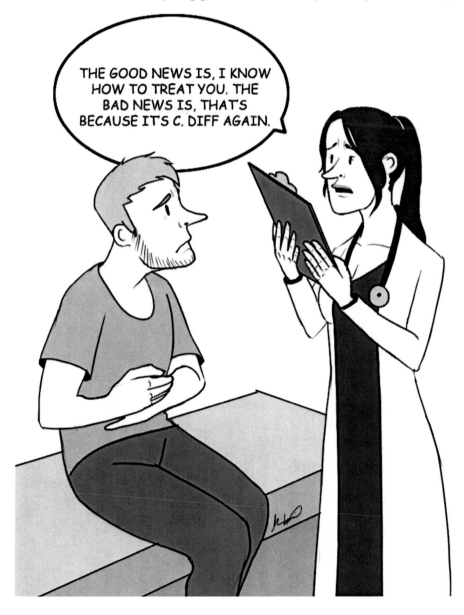

THE GOOD NEWS IS, I KNOW HOW TO TREAT YOU. THE BAD NEWS IS, THAT'S BECAUSE IT'S C. DIFF AGAIN.

but perhaps with an even longer taper.

Regardless of how your doctor chooses to move forward, you will likely be feeling pretty hopeless and scared at this point, thinking that you're always going to be suffering from this horrible disease. But you won't be. The general belief amongst doctors is that the tapered-pulsed dosing method (using vancomycin or some other antibiotic) cures everyone eventually. We should also add that the research supports this belief[14]. It may take longer than usual, and it will certainly not be fun, but essentially everyone gets rid of C. diff eventually. Chris, one of the authors of this book, had four recurrences of C. diff after his initial infection, and a second tapered-pulse eventually got rid of it for good. His last tapered-pulse went on for about three months, but it worked.

This is never going to end!!!
Every patient with recurrent C. diff thinks this at some point during his or her illness. Some will think it every day. This is only natural, given the unpredictable nature of recurrent C. diff, but it is almost always false. Permanently recurring C. diff is so rare as to be something doctors don't even think about. You are going to get over this infection, although it will take patience, persistence, and a bit of luck. We say luck only because it's hard to predict which round of treatment will work for you, but we have absolute confidence that one of them will. Try to bring some humor to the situation. Stock up on magazines to read in the bathroom (but leave them in the bathroom!). And if you find yourself feeling really hopeless, seek out some professional help for your mood.

Alternative Therapies for Recurrent C. diff

While the tapered-pulse described above has become the treatment of choice for those with recurrent C. diff, there are other treatments out there. We're listing them here because your doctor may suggest them as an alternative or a complement to the standard therapies. Likewise, you may wish to mention them to your doctor if you feel your current treatment isn't working as well as you'd like. Keep in mind however, that we strongly believe that the tapered-pulse is the best treatment for recurrent C. diff, and we wouldn't encourage any patient to give up on that approach just because it didn't work the first time. Rather, we would encourage patients to add some mixture of these complementary treatments to a second or third tapered-pulse, rather than replacing it.

Antibiotic "Chasers"

A number of doctors are having success in treating recurrent C. difficile by following treatment with vancomycin or Flagyl with a "chaser" of another antibiotic. Many doctors who use the "chaser" approach like to give rifaximin after a tapered-pulse of vancomycin similar to the one listed above. Rifaximin is a drug similar in behavior and treatment success to vancomycin, but for some reason, administering rifaximin after vancomycin seems particularly effective in treating recurrent C. diff. In one small study, seven of eight patients given a rifaximin chaser after standard treatment with vancomycin were cured of C. diff symptoms and experienced no recurrences. The eighth had an equally positive outcome after one more round of rifaximin[15]. It may be that C. diff spores are tricked into hatching by changing up the medicines attacking them, but at the moment, doctor's aren't sure why this technique works well. More study in this area is needed.

Stool Transplants

While you might normally laugh in the face of a doctor suggesting you ingest someone else's poop, once you've suffered through a few rounds of C. diff, you'll be willing to consider anything. Stool transplants rest on the theory that C. diff bacteria can only thrive in a human gut that has been emptied of its normal, healthy, and competitive flora[16]. Since those antibiotics you took wiped out your own gut flora, a stool transplant seeks to replace it with someone else's. This technique is much more popular in Europe than it is in the U.S., but more and more doctors are adopting the technique here.

A typical stool transplant begins with stool freshly donated from a heavily-screened, disease-free donor. That stool is then washed multiple times with sterile water, and the resulting filtrate is introduced into the patient's gut via x-ray-guided nasogastric tube, or via enema or during colonoscopy. The patient has typically been prepped with a short round of vancomycin to suppress the levels of C. diff in their guts. After this short procedure, the patient is free to go about their business and will hopefully return almost immediately to a pre-C. diff state as the donated bacterial flora quickly multiplies to fill up their gut within hours or days.

As gross as it might sound, stool transplants have been highly effective in the admittedly small patient populations in which they have been attempted. In a small, uncontrolled study, 15 of 18 patients who had suffered from recurrent C. diff were cured by stool trans-plants[17]. There are more and more small-scale studies like these that are showing fecal transplant to be a promising alternative for C. diff patients who are tired of the seemingly endless cycle of antibiotics - C. diff - antibiotics – and more C. diff. However, given the potential dangers involved (even if your stool donor comes back clean, be aware that communicable diseases might be missed on tests) and the usual success of the tapered-pulse method, the authors of the book advocate for the safer route. There are currently no large-scale studies validating the benefits of stool transplant over the risks, and the tapered-pulse looks like the best way to go for the majority of recurrent C. diff sufferers at the moment. However, it is something to talk about with your doctor if you have relapsed multiple times and are ready for something more drastic. If you see a stool transplant as your last, best hope to get over C. diff, at the very least make sure your donor has been screened for communicable diseases and use a doctor who is familiar with the procedure. You don't want to trade C. diff for hepatitis or some other communicable disease you'll have for the rest of your life.

Probiotics

Remember back in Chapters One and Two, when we talked about using probiotics to prevent and treat initial infections of C. diff? Well, it should come as no surprise that doctors also use them to help break the cycle of recurrent C. diff. the thinking goes, if we can get some healthy, helpful microorganisms in there while we're killing the C. diff, then we stand a better chance of your gut getting fully colonized with a healthy flora before C. diff can build up its numbers enough to attack you again. Does it work? Well, the numbers are honestly a bit muddled on the effectiveness of probiotics in preventing and treating

Antibodies and Antigens: Antibodies are the blood hounds of your immune system. They're large proteins that float around in the body, sniffing around at everything they see. When they find an invader they've seen before (like a cold virus), or one that they don't recognize (like a C. diff bacterium), they glom onto that invader protein and label it for destruction at the hands of the immune system.

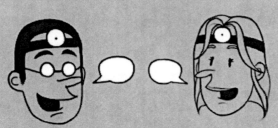

C. diff, but in at least one study, patients with a history of recurrent C. diff had significantly fewer future recurrences if they were given the probiotic yeast Saccharomyces boulardii at the same time[18]. Yeasts are fungi (like mushrooms), not bacteria, and they may be particularly useful as probiotics because they are not killed by the antibiotics that are going after the C. diff.

Research on probiotic Lactobacillus bacteria are also a bit muddled, with some research suggesting they help prevent recurrence[19], and some research finding no positive effect[20]. Most doctors agree that probiotics alone have little hope of ending recurrent C. diff and should be paired with some other therapy, like antibiotics.

For the most part, treatment with probiotics is considered fairly harmless, but as we mentioned earlier, there have been cases of both fungal and bacterial probiotics infecting immune-compromised individuals, so we always recommending consulting with your doctor before beginning probiotics. They can also be quite expensive, and there is often a "breaking in" period of a couple of weeks, when they can cause gas and bloating until your gut and they adapt to one another.

Intravenous Immunoglobulin and Antibody Therapies

As mentioned above, there appears to be a direct connection between the strength of a patient's immune response to C. diff and the potential for infection and recurrence. Realizing that our own bodies are the best infection fighters we have at our disposal, some doctors have tried boosting patients' immune responses to C. diff by injecting them with a substance called intravenous immunoglobulin, an immune booster that helps make our bodies more aware of the invaders in the system. Specifically, doctors use immunoglobulin that contains an anti-toxin to C. diff toxin A. Introducing these anti-toxins into infected patients' bodies has been shown to boost those patients' response to C. diff and has led to subsequent

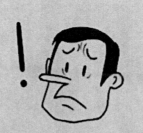

I can't afford this right now! With all the trips to the doctor, the tests, and the medications, getting sick with C. diff is as hard on the wallet as it is on the body. If you don't have insurance and pay for drugs out of pocket, C. diff can be devastating. A long taper of Vancomycin pills can easily cost in the thousands of dollars (it's not unusual for a 10-day run to cost between $1,500 and $2,000). Consider asking around for a pharmacy that will provide liquid Vancomycin instead. Liquid Vancomycin (typically given in IVs) is comparable to the pill form when take orally and is much cheaper (sometimes as cheap as $100 for a 30-day supply, though costs can be higher than that).

resolution of the infection[21].

Working off the same theory as that advocated above, doctors have also given C. diff patients a concentrate of antibody-rich immune protein compounds isolated from the milk of cows that have been immunized to C. diff bacteria and toxins. Of 16 patients (nine of whom had a history of recurring C. diff) treated with this protein concentrate after a standard run of antibiotics, none suffered another episode of C. diff diarrhea during a 333 day follow-up period[22]. Results like these suggest that our best weapon against C. diff is our own bodies, and that if we can teach our bodies how to fight C. diff better, most patients will kill off the infection on their own.

Sequestrants

Just as sequestrants are used to treat initial infections of C. diff, resins like cholestrymine and colestipol may be used to help end the cycle of recurrent C. diff. As a reminder, sequestrants are given orally to C. diff patients to bind the C. diff toxins in their guts and carry them out of their systems. In at least one small, uncontrolled study, 11 recurrent-C. diff patients treated with both tapered vancomycin and sequestrants were cured and C. diff-free after six weeks of follow-up[23]. As we mentioned in Chapter Two, sequestrants can also bind any medicines in your system (like the antibiotics being used to treat C. diff) and render them inactive. So, if your doctor does prescribe a sequestrant, make sure you take it as far from the time you are taking your medicines as you can.

Some sequestrants in development (e.g. Tolevamer) do such a good job of binding C. diff toxins that they are almost as effective in ending C. diff disease as the antibiotics themselves, and they have a markedly lower recurrence rate[24].

If All Else Fails

In those extremely rare cases where the cycle of recurrence cannot be stopped, patients have been kept on a low dose of vancomycin (125mg daily or every other day) permanently. This is a horribly expensive treatment, and therefore trying for the patient on a number of levels, but it can work if nothing else does. It is also not ideal given the increased possibility that the C. diff in this patient may develop a resistance to the vancomycin (although this has not been seen as of yet). We want to reiterate how incredibly rare this situation is; you will be hard pressed to find a doctor who has ever heard of such a patient, much less met one. The vast majority of patients with recurrent C. diff are cured within a few weeks to a few months, and the tiny minority that won't be cured for over a year will eventually be cured.

We also want to mention here that it is possible that your primary care physician will not be familiar with some of these lesser known treatments for C. diff. And while an infectious disease specialist or a gastroenterologist is likely to know about the pros and cons of these alternative treatments, keep in mind that they rarely need to use them — for the vast majority of patients, the tapered-pulse will do the trick.

The Dos and Don'ts of Talking with Your Doctor

We want to spend a few moments talking about how you and your doctor can communicate to your best advantage. For recurrent C. diff patients, this is a particularly important issue because you're going to be talking to your doctor a lot over the next few weeks or months, and you want that communication to be productive. So let's talk about some Dos and Don'ts for effective patient-doctor communication.

DO educate yourself. Read this book. Read any articles that sound interesting to you, but **DON'T** try to be your own doctor and **DON'T** swamp your doctor with a pile of the latest research on *C. difficile* treatment. Instead, you might say something like, "I have read that some doctors have had success using antibiotic chasers after a tapered-pulse treatment. What do you think of that method?"

DO find a way to easily communicate with your doctor, but **DON'T** abuse that communication path. If you find a doctor who is kind enough to share their e-mail or cell phone number with you, rejoice, but make sure you don't abuse that privilege. Doctors are among the busiest professionals out there these days, and you will quickly lose any goodwill yours has extended to you if you call them after every bowel movement. Instead, agree on a plan of action when you meet with them, and save the personal calls for true emergencies. For example, you might come up with a plan like, "I'm going to take the Flagyl until Thursday. If I have diarrhea on Friday, I'm going to wait to call you and see if it subsides over the weekend. If it isn't gone by Monday, I'm going to take this test kit you've given me and do another stool test. If it gets really bad and scary any time over the weekend, I'm going to call you. Is that what you want me to do?"

DO seek a second opinion, but **DON'T** go behind your doctor's back. If you feel like you're not getting the best care you can from your doctor, seek a second opinion. Try to speak to a specialist or just another practitioner. Really, it's okay. A good doctor will know that you're just looking at all your options. But no one likes to be talked about behind their back. So respect your doctor as a professional and a fellow adult and tell them, "I hope you won't be offended, but I'm nervous as hell about this whole thing, and I'm going to talk to a specialist about it just to calm my nerves. I hope this won't impact our doctor-patient relationship, which I very much appreciate."

DO question your doctor, professionally and respectfully.

DO trust that they have your best interests at heart, and while they are only human, they are doing their best to heal you.

DO expect to be treated with kindness and respect as a patient, an adult, and educated person. And if you are not being treated as such, consider finding another doctor who will treat you with the kindness and respect you deserve.

DO thank doctors while they are working with you *and* after you've gotten better. It's a common decency which they so rarely hear these days.

Notes – Chapter Three

1. Maroo S. & Lamont J.T. (2006) Recurrent *Clostridium difficile*. Gastroenterology, 130:1311.

2. Arroyo, L.G., Kruth, S.A., Willey, B.M., Staempfli, H.R., Low, D.E., & Weese, J.S. (2005). PCR ribotyping of *Clostridium difficile* isolates originating from human and animal sources. Journal of Medical Microbiology, 54(2): 163, and Borriello, S.P., Honour, P., Turner, T., & Barclay, F. (1983). Household pets as a potential reservoir for *Clostridium difficile* infection. Journal of Clinical Pathology, 36: 84.

3. Segarra-Newnham, M. (2007). Probiotics for *Clostridium difficile*–Associated Diarrhea: Focus on *Lactobacillus rhamnosus* GG and Saccharomyces boulardii. The Annals of Pharmacotherapy, 41: 1212.

4. Segarra-Newnham, 2007.

5. McFarland, L.V., Surawicz, C.M., Rubin, M., Fekety, R., Elmer, G.W., & Greenberg, R.N. (1999), Recurrent *Clostridium difficile* Disease: Epidemiology and Clinical Characteristics. Infection Control and Hospital Epidemiology, 20(1): 43.

6. Peláez, T., Alcalá, L., Alonso, R., Rodríguez-Créixems, M., Garcia-Lechuz, J.M., & Bouza, E. (2002). Reassessment of *Clostridium difficile* susceptibility to metronidazole and vancomycin. Antimicrobial Agents and Chemotherapy, 46(6): 1647.

7. Maroo and Lamont, 2006.

8. Wilcox, M.H., Fawley, W.N., Settle, C.D. & Davidson, A. (1998). Recurrence of symptoms in *Clostridium difficile* infection – relapse or reinfection?. Journal of Hospital Infections, 38: 93.

9. Johal, S.S., Lambert, C.P., Hammond, J., James, P.D., Borriello, S.P., & Mahida, Y.R. (2004). Colonic IgA producing cells and macrophages are reduced in recurrent and non-recurrent *Clostridium difficile*-associated diarrhoea. Journal of Clinical Pathology, 57: 973.

10. Kyne, L., Warny, M., Qamar, A., & Kelly, C.P. (2000). Asymptomatic carriage of *Clostridium difficile* and serum levels of IgG antibody against toxin A. The New England Journal of Medicine, 342(6): 390.

11. Sanchez, J.L., Gerding, D.N., Olson, M.M. & Johnson, S. (1999).

Metronidazole susceptibility in *Clostridium difficile* isolates re-covered from cases of C.difficile-associated disease treatment failures and successes. Anaerobe 5: 201.

12. McFarland, L.V., Elmer, G.W. & Surawicz, C.M. (2002). Breaking the cycle: treatment strategies for 163 cases of recurrent *Clostridium difficile* disease. American Journal of Gastroenterology, 97: 1769.

13. Kelly, C.P. & LaMont, J.T. (2008). *Clostridium difficile* – More difficult than ever. The New England Journal of Medicine, 359(18): 1932.

14. Maroo and LaMont, 2006 and Tedesco, F.J., Gordon, D., & Fortson, W.C. (1985). Approach to patients with multiple relatpses of antibi-otic-associated pseudomembranous colitis. American Journal of Gastroenterology, 80: 867.

15. Johnson, S., Schriever, C., Galang, M., Kelly, C.P., & Gerding, D.N. (2007). Interruption of recurrent *Clostridium difficile*-associated diarrhea episodes by serial therapy with vancomycin and rifaxi-min. Clinical Infectious Diseases, 44: 846.

16. Tvede, M. & Rask-Madsen, J. (1989). Bacteriotherapy for chronic relapsing *Clostridium difficile* diarrhea in six patients. The Lancet, 333(8648): 1156.

17. Aas, J., Gessert, C.E., & Bakken, J.S. (2003). Recurrent *Clostridium difficile* colitis: Case series involving 18 patients treated with donor stool administered via a nasogastric tube. Clinical Infectious Diseases, 36: 580.

18. McFarland, L.V., Surawicz, C.M., Greenberg, R.N., Fekety, R., Elmer, G.W., Moyer, K.A., Melcher, S.A., Bowen, K.E., Cox, J.L., Noorani, Z., Harrington, G., Rubin, M., & Greenwald, D. (1994). A randomized placebo-controlled trial of Saccharomyces boulardii in combina-tion with standard antibiotics for *Clostridium difficile* disease. Jour-nal of the American Medical Association, 272: 518.

19. Gorbach, S.L., Chang, T.W., & Goldin, B. (1987). Successful treat-ment of relapsing *Clostridium difficile* colitis with Lactobacillus GG. The Lancet, 26: 1519.

20. Thomas, M.R., Litin, S.C., Osmon, D.R., Corr, A.P., Weaver, A.L., & Lohse, C.M. (2001). Lack of effect of *lactobacillus* GG on antibi-otic-associated diarrhea: A randomized, placebo-controlled trial. Mayo Clinic Proceedings, 76(9): 883.

21. Wilcox, M.H. (2004). Descriptive study of intravenous immunoglob-

ulin for the treatment of recurrent *Clostridium difficile* diarrhoea. Journal of Antimicrobial Chemotherapy, 53: 882 and Leung, D.Y., Kelly, C.P., Boguniewicz, M., Pothoulakis, C., LaMont, J.T. & Flores, A. (1991). Treatment with intravenously administered gamma globulin of chronic relapsing colitis inducted by *Clostridium difficile* toxin. Journal of Pediatrics, 118: 633.

22.   Van Dissel, J.T., de Groot, N., Hensgens, C.M.H., Numan, S., Kuijper, E.J., Veldkamp, P., & van't Woot, J. (2005). Bovine antibody-enriched whey to aid in the prevention of a relapse of *Clostridium difficile* associated diarrhoea: Preclinical and preliminary clinical data. Journal of Medical Microbiology, 54: 197.

23.   Tedesco, F.J. (1982). Pseudomembranous colitis: Pathogenesis and therapy. Medical Clinics of North America, 66: 655.

24.   Monaghan, T., Boswell, T., & Mahida, Y.R. (2008). Recent advances in *Clostridium difficile*-associated disease. Gut, 57: 850.

Chapter Four
The Aftermath of C. difficile

Despite what your own experience has been up to this point, C. diff is not a chronic disease; it is an acute one. Chronic diseases are permanent diseases for the patients who have them, or they are of such long duration and uncertain prospects that they might as well be permanent. Heart disease, diabetes, muscular sclerosis — these are all chronic diseases. Recurrent C. diff may last many months, and because of this, and the seeming uncertainty of avoiding a relapse, it may seem chronic — but it is not. You will get over it, typically in a few weeks, sometimes in a few months. However, C. diff can wreak quite a bit of damage on your system, both physically and emotionally, and it can take months, or even years, for your body and mind to return to normal. Rarely, C. diff patients may even find that their guts are never quite the same again. Because of this, we wanted to dedicate at least a chapter of this book to life after C. diff.

Additionally, we want to spend some time in this chapter talking about the worst case scenario: when C. diff claims a loved one. When writing this book, we started with the assumption that most of the people buying it would be those who were suffering from recurrent C. diff. As a rule, C. diff is not fatal for recurrent C. diff sufferers. It affects their quality of life, their happiness, and their overall health and well being, but if C. diff didn't kill you the first time around, it's very, very, very unlikely that it will ever kill you. Having said that, C. diff does kill — from 1999–2004, C. diff was reported as a cause of death for 20,642 Americans[1], and this number is likely a conservative one,

Other problems from C. diff: Like many diseases, C. diff hurts you in multiple ways. You already know that C. diff can damage your guts, but there's evidence that C. diff infection also can result in kidney injury[2], and some will go on to develop temporary arthritis that seems to be a reaction to the bug[3].

since C. diff is often a contributing factor in deaths that are attributed to other causes. However, the vast majority of people who die from C. diff are "high-risk" patients: the elderly, those with compromised immune systems (e.g., from active AIDS) or guts (as in those with Inflammatory Bowel Disease), and those who are already suffering from other major illnesses.

This chapter may not give you the peace of mind you're looking for, but after reading it, we hope you'll have a better idea about how to move forward from C. diff and find that peace of mind for yourself.

90 Days to freedom

While there is no hard and fast rule for declaring a C. diff patient "re-covered," most doctors agree that if you make it 70-90 days without a C. diff recurrence, then you are very, very likely in the clear. Friendly bacteria will begin to re-colonize your gut almost immediately after you go off antibiotics, and after just a couple of weeks, your gut flora will begin to look like it did before you took antibiotics. And remember, the vast majority of C. diff recurrences occur within a month of ending antibiotics. Still, those in the C. diff community give it 90 days, just to be doubly certain. Unfortunately, because of their past experiences, re-current C. diff sufferers will find the 90-day waiting period an agonizing series of false alarms (and sometimes not-so-false alarms) and stressful expectation.

For those of you in the middle of your 90 days now, please take these words to heart: You are going to get over this disease. Perma-nently recurring C. diff is extraordinarily rare. For all practical purposes, no one has this disease forever. Now, this may be your golden 90 days, and it may not. You may have another recurrence and need to try something different: perhaps a longer taper, perhaps a new antibiotic – but take heart, one of these 90 days is going to stick.

Even if this is your golden 90 days, and you are free and clear of C. diff already, it may be a rough three months. There are no exact numbers on this, but anecdotally, doctors estimate that between 4% and 32% of patients will suffer from post-infectious irritable bowel syndrome (PI-IBS) for some time after a bacterial infection[4]. We'll talk about IBS in a moment, but its implication for your 90 days is this: IBS can mimic C. diff in almost every way. While suffering from bouts of IBS,

102

Will I always be susceptible to C. diff? Many C. diff sufferers worry that they will always be at risk of getting C. diff if they take another antibiotic in the near or distant future. Anecdotally, many patients report that their doctors confirm this fear, telling them things like, "Now that you've got C. diff in you, you'll always need to be careful." While we can understand this fear, we can find no support for it in the medical literature. To our knowledge, no one has actually tracked future susceptibility of ex-C. diff patients to future infections. Studies on long-term carriage of C. diff suggest that almost all patients have flushed the bug out of their system after only a couple of months[5]. While we advise everyone to avoid antibiotics unless they really need them, we don't see any reason to avoid or even fear antibiotics when they are really needed. Odds are very good that you will never have C. diff again.

you can have watery diarrhea, mucous in your stools, cramps, bloating, and all the misery you associate with C. diff. IBS should NOT lead to blood in your stools (unless you have hemorrhoids, which is entirely possible, even likely, with IBS); blood in your stools, with diarrhea, is a good indication that your C. diff may be back, and that you need a C. diff test. Chris, one of the authors of this book, suffered from repeated bouts of IBS during his golden 90 days (and long after, unfortunately). He was constantly convinced his C. diff was coming back, only to have the diarrhea and cramps dissipate after a few days and turn out not to be C. diff after all.

On the C. diff support forums at www.cdiffsupport.com, the veteran contributors constantly preach the "Three Day Rule." When you are having what you think might be a C. diff recurrence, suffer through it for at least three days before getting a test or going on more antibiotics. More often than not, the alarm will turn out to be a false one, and going on antibiotics would have been a mistake. Chris made this horrible mistake at least once during his five bouts with C. diff. About a week after a round of vancomycin, he had a bout of IBS, but thinking it was C. diff, he started to take another round of antibiotics before getting his test results back. All three test samples came back negative for C. diff, but Chris was already on the antibiotics and decided to finish the round, leading to another recurrence of C. diff two weeks later. Don't make this mistake. Don't panic, trust your doctor, trust the C. diff tests, and have faith that you will beat this beast eventually.

Irritable Bowel Syndrome — The gift that keeps on giving

Congratulations, you made it through your golden 90 days, and your odds of having another C. diff recurrence are close to zero. But here you are, six months after your last round of antibiotics, and your guts still don't seem right. You're still going to the bathroom multiple times a day, often have diarrhea, and suffer from abdominal pain that strikes without warning. Repeated stool tests have come back negative for C. diff, and your doctor is convinced that you are over the bug. You're deeply tired of living this way and wish your doctor could offer you something more than the diagnosis that patients in this situation invariably get: Irritable Bowel Syndrome.

As we said above, doctors estimate that between 4% and 32% of patients will develop irritable bowel syndrome (or IBS) for some time after any bacterial or parasitic infection. At least one study has looked specifically at IBS rates following C. diff infection and found good news: of 23 patients with C. diff, eight exhibited some degree of IBS

IBS vs. IBD: There are so many acronyms that doctors use, and it doesn't help that half of them sound exactly the same! Remember that IBS stands for Irritable Bowel Syndrome. IBS is a disorder common after a gut infection, and can be associated with either diarrhea or constipation, or both – but never with visible damage to the gut. IBS is commonly treated with medicines meant to improve gut function.

IBD stands for Inflammatory Bowel Disease and is an autoimmune disorder of the gut that results in chronic inflammation, ulcers, scarring and abscesses. IBD must be treated with medications that modulate the function of the immune system, like steroids.

For the C. diff patient, remember that C. diff doesn't cause IBD (though it can cause a flare-up of someone's IBD), whereas C. diff can result in IBS that lasts for a few months to a few years, and in rare cases, permanently.

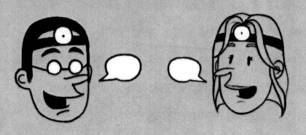

directly following resolution of the infection, while the other 15 were symptom-free. But three months later, only one of the initial 23 patients still had IBS problems; the others were doing just fine[6]. The author also notes that that one last patient with IBS had particularly bad C. diff. This suggests that C. diff has a lower rate of IBS following infection than other gut bugs, but that longer, tougher C. diff may increase your chances of things not working quite right for a while after infection.

For those unlucky few who do have long-term IBS following C. diff (in which case it is called post-infectious irritable bowel syndrome, or PI-IBS), their problems aren't over, even after they've gotten rid of the bug. For months, perhaps years afterwards, they will suffer from frequent, potentially loose stools, stomach pain and unease, urgency, and generally unhappy guts. While IBS is a fairly safe diagnosis for these sorts of symptoms after an infection, a good gastroenterologist will want to make sure there isn't something scarier going on that could be mimicking the symptoms of IBS (like cancer or inflammatory bowel disease). Don't get too worried about that last sentence. Intestinal cancers and inflammatory bowel disease are comparatively rare. IBS is all too common. There are some estimates that up to 35% of Americans will suffer from IBS some time in their lives.

Doctors put IBS in three categories. In IBS-diarrhea predominant (IBS-D), diarrhea and frequent stools are the distinguishing factors. In IBS-constipation predominant (IBS-C), episodes are characterized by constipation and low frequency of stools. In IBS-alternating (IBS-A), patients flip flop between diarrhea and constipation. Post-infectious IBS tends to be of the diarrheal variety, but not always.

The good news is that doctors are very convinced that IBS doesn't hurt you. In fact, IBS is called a "functional disorder" because it only seems to affect the function of the guts. When doctors look for damage to the intestines in IBS patients, they rarely find anything. The best they can do is show some inflammation at the cellular level in some IBS patients. We can also take some solace in the fact that the prognosis for PI-IBS is better than that for chronic, non-infection-related IBS. The majority of PI-IBS sufferers will see an improvement or cessation of symptoms within three years. The bad news is that because it is a functional disorder, and a poorly understood one at that, it is very likely that the best your doctor will be able to do is manage the symptoms of IBS and hope fervently that you get better over time.

IBS is a medical issue deserving its own book (and there are a few out there that may be helpful), so we are not going to be able to do it justice here. However, in the next couple of pages, we're going to address some of the most common and the most promising treatments for IBS, since we know that a portion of the people reading this book will suffer from it. For the most part, IBS treatment falls into three categories: diet, stress management, and drug therapy.

Diet

Most IBS patients have a list of "trigger foods" that, if eaten, are more likely to result in an IBS attack than other foods. Trigger foods vary from individual to individual, but all IBS sufferers would do well to avoid GI irritants like coffee (both caffeinated and decaffeinated), alcohol, sodas and artificial sweeteners. Moderation is generally the key when making daily food choices for IBS. Avoid meals that are particularly

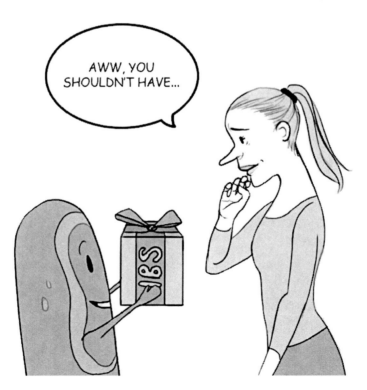

fatty (French fries are a classic IBS trigger) or have lots of insoluble fiber, like salads and raw vegetables. Gas-producing foods like garlic, beans and cabbage may also cause problems for some, as IBS patients tend to be more aware of, and more sensitive to, the pain and discomfort of bloating when compared to non-IBS sufferers.

Each IBS patient is unique and will have unique dietary needs and tolerances. Rather than cut all possible triggers out of your diet wholesale, keep a food and symptom log at every meal, and after a week or two, you'll have a better idea of which meals are tolerable, and which will keep you chained to the toilet the next day. Moderation is also the key here; big, heavy meals are much more likely to trigger IBS attacks than smaller, lighter meals scattered throughout the day.

Hypnotherapy and Stress Reduction Therapy

Have you ever been in a particularly nerve-wracking situation and felt a sudden need to go to the bathroom, a need that wasn't there a moment ago? Most people have, and it's no surprise. This instinct goes all the way back to our most basic fight-or-flight response. As humans were evolving, one of the physical behaviors that we developed was the voiding of one's bladder and bowels in moments of extreme stress. Many animals do this, in fact. We can only guess at why we do this. Perhaps it was a good way to "lighten the load" if you needed to run from an angry wooly mammoth, and of course it leaves an unpleasant surprise behind for anything that might be trying to eat you. This intimate connection between our bowels and our stress management system has stayed largely intact despite the rarity of wooly mammoth attacks for modern humans. Now, we find that the relatively mild but

In the spring of 2008, my family and I went to lunch at a local restaurant. A few hours later, I began to feel sick and had several bouts of diarrhea. I assumed it was food poisoning and didn't worry about it. I had recently given birth to my daughter and figured I just needed to take better care of myself.

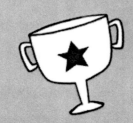

After a few days of feeling ill and having diarrhea five to six times a day, I went to see my doctor. She ran several tests and could not find anything wrong, but she prescribed a short course of an antibiotic anyway. After completing the antibiotics I still felt sick and the diarrhea continued. Not seeing any improvement I returned to the doctor. That's when I was diagnosed with C. diff and was put on Flagyl for 10 days. The diarrhea stopped and I began to feel better.

I was devastated when I relapsed shortly after going off that first round of Flagyl, and I was given Flagyl again, this time for 14 days. The frequent diarrhea stopped after that, but every few weeks I would have an episode or two and would be convinced it was C. diff again. I'm apparently one of those people who "carries" C. diff around, as I would test positive for C. diff even it I wasn't having symptoms.

My fear of C. diff coming back ruled my life. I did not trust that my home was free of C-diff spores and began to obsess about personal hygiene. I got in the habit of washing my hands constantly and handling my food with napkins, so as to not re-infect myself. For a long time I limited my diet to simple carbohydrates and dairy, things I considered "safe". Eating out was no longer an option, as I did not trust any establishment to properly handle their food.

If you let it, C. diff can take over your life in ways you never imagined. I have put the episode behind me and am starting to enjoy food and life again. Therapy and a lot of self-determination to live my life again have brought me a long way. I hate what C. diff did to me and hope that other C. diff sufferers who read this will NOT follow in my footsteps. C. diff is bad enough physically; don't let it cripple you emotionally as well.

Victoria O, Tustin, CA

more constant stressors of daily life can wreak havoc on our guts, particularly for those of us with IBS.

Despite what many doctors used to think, stress does not cause IBS, but it can exacerbate it, and is more often than not the trigger for an IBS attack. So, it should come as no surprise that doctors try to manage IBS symptoms by addressing the amount of stress in their patient's lives. This may mean identifying sources of stress in our lives and removing them – perhaps finding a new job if our old one is driving us batty. It may also mean using different forms of psychological therapy to address and mediate the ways that we deal with our stressors.

There are many forms of psycho-therapy, or "talk therapy," and a number of them hold promise for dealing with IBS. The most promising form (and the most interesting, we think) is hypnotherapy. In hypnotherapy, the therapist helps the patient achieve a level of deep relaxation, and then uses that relaxed state as a place to connect the patient with his or her subconscious bodily functions. In the case of IBS hypnotherapy, the therapist uses suggestion and imagery to help the deeply relaxed patient learn to slow down and relax the speed at which their guts process food. Slower, calmer guts equal less bowel urgency and less bowel discomfort for IBS-D patients. Should you suffer from IBS-C, your hypnotist would work with you to speed up the rate of your guts.

Drugs

Most gastroenterologists will have medications in their toolbox for treating IBS. Some of the most commonly used IBS-D medications are tricyclic antidepressants like amitriptyline. Tricyclics help regulate the amount of natural human hormone called serotonin in the gut and brain. Serotonin is key in regulating mood and gut function, and seems to not function quite right in many patients with IBS. Tricyclics are also inherently constipating, and this can be helpful for patients with diarrhea-predominant IBS (the most common post-infectious IBS).

Tricyclics represent just one of many classes of drugs that have been shown to improve symptoms of IBS and the resulting quality of life for the patient. Don't give up on your doctor because the first drug they prescribed didn't help you. Your body is unique, and what works for someone else may not work for you. It is not unusual for an IBS patient to try two or three different drugs before finding one that works wonders for their guts.

Antibiotics

Yes, you read that header right. There is an increasingly popular theory that a percentage of IBS symptoms are caused by an overgrowth of bacteria in the small intestine. Not surprisingly, doctors who subscribe to this theory generally try to treat IBS with antibiotics. This solution does work for a number of IBS sufferers, but as you have likely already surmised, this kind of treatment carries with it the risk of another C. diff infection. It is therefore not a popular one with those recovering from C. diff. If your IBS is so bad that you're willing to try antibiotics again, we recommend the book, *A New IBS Solution*, by Mark Pimentel (published by Health Point Press, 2005). Without going into details about his methodology, suffice it to say that Dr. Pimentel is one of the pioneers of this method of treating IBS. While we might argue with the scope of his claims about the efficacy of this brand of treatment, we do believe that antibiotic therapy does offer some hope for a percentage of IBS sufferers. Reading his book will prepare you for a conversation with your gastroenterologist about trying this treatment. Keep in mind, as we always say, whether you've had C. diff or not, every usage of antibiotics comes with some risk of C. diff infection, however small.

Emotional Recovery

C. diff is a scary, scary disease. For many it is not the severity of the illness which is frightening (although it can be), it is instead the randomness with which C. diff strikes. Particularly for those with recurrent C. diff, there is a constant hope that the current bout will be your last one, and the ever-present fear that you'll never be free of the disease. For those first few weeks after the infection has been seemingly cured, every stomach pain brings with it fear and unease, and every trip to the bathroom is an exercise in anticipation. "Is this the time it comes back?" It can take a very long time to shake that fear and accept that C. diff is gone, this time, for good.

Like other long-term diseases, C. diff can be a real test of a relationship. Because it is such an unknown disease, spouses, friends, and family may be relatively unsympathetic to someone who they think "just has the runs." If you are the C. diff patient, consider sharing this book with those who aren't "getting it." If you are a spouse or a friend reading this book, please trust us when we tell you that your loved one has a very serious disease. It's true that it's unlikely to kill them, but we can tell you from personal experience that they are probably in the most pain and discomfort they've ever been in, and they have a right to be scared, worried, and miserable. When trying to describe the ordeal of C. diff to someone new, Chris, one of the authors of this book, would use the old joke: "first I was afraid I was going to die, then I was afraid I wasn't going to die." It was still a joke, but far less of one than it had been before C. diff.

Some who have suffered from C. diff will develop an anxious fear of germs, diarrhea, and disease in general. For some this anxiety will be mild, short-lived, and something they might laugh about later in life. For others it will blossom into a full-blown anxiety disorder that limits what they eat, how they live, and how much they enjoy life. Washing your hands after using the bathroom, changing a baby's diaper, and before cooking or eating is good sanitation. Washing your hands every ten minutes, avoiding perfectly safe foods, and never going to restaurants is not good sanitation, it's just anxiety. Be on the alert for the emotional scars of C. diff, and seek medical treatment for them just as you would seek treatment for the physical scars. Modern psychological medicine considers post-traumatic stress (which this certainly seems to be a form of) and anxiety to be very treatable diseases. If you find yourself obsessing about the possible return of C. diff many months after your infections have stopped, then it's high time to talk to your family doctor about it.

Even if you don't think of yourself as someone who needs medical help, you might benefit from a community of other sufferers. We highly recommend checking out the forums at www.cdiffsupport. com. Here you'll find others who share your experiences, your pain, your hopes, and your understanding of this nasty disease. As we've mentioned before, because it is a "bathroom disease," C. diff can be especially isolating. Getting wisdom from other sufferers, and sharing your own wisdom, can go a long way towards reducing your anxieties.

How does someone die of C. diff?

C. diff kills in two primary ways. In some cases, the diarrhea from C. diff is so frequent, and so severe, that the dehydration it causes taxes the body beyond recovery. This dehydration might be tolerable in an otherwise healthy patient, particularly if they are receiving fluids, nutrients, and medicine via an intravenous drip, but in an elderly patient, in someone who is very sick with some other disease, or in someone with

extremely severe C. diff, the patient may become overwhelmed by this dehydration and die.

In other cases, the amount of C. diff toxins in the gut becomes so high that the cells in the walls of the large intestine are poisoned to death and stop functioning. This very serious scenario is called "paralytic illeus." Paralytic illeus is particularly bad because it is self-reinforcing. Toxins build up in the gut, causing it to stop working and therefore to stop clearing the toxins out of the gut, allowing them to build up even more. Anti-diarrheal drugs like Imodium, which further suppress the gut's natural contractions, can make this condition worse, and are thus not advised in patients with severe C. diff as much as they might like a break from the diarrhea. Ultimately, this chain of events can lead to a very rare but very scary situation called "toxic megacolon." In toxic megacolon the patient's colon dilates massively in a matter of hours. Fever and shock often accompany the dilation, which can lead to a tear in the colon wall if not dealt with immediately. In this very rare situation, doctors have little choice but to attempt a partial or complete colonectomy (surgical removal of the large intestine). Even if they are able to do this, the patients' chances of dying after the operation are still frighteningly high, upwards of 20-30%.

We want to emphasize again that death from C. diff is relatively rare. Research puts the overall percentage of C. diff deaths at about 2.3% of all cases, and at about 6.1% for those deeply ill patients in intensive care units[7]. These are very low numbers, and these percentages are likely biased towards older, more fragile patients, and those with other diseases. To those of you who have lost a loved one to C. diff, you have our deepest and most sincere sympathy; we know these percentages do nothing to assuage your grief. We also know that there are exceptions to every rule and C. diff may have claimed the life of a healthy loved one in the prime of their life, despite our reassurances above. It's hard for us to imagine how upset and angry you must feel. In the next section we do our meager best to answer some of the questions you must surely have about why your loved one died.

To those of you who have not lost a loved one, but are afraid of dying yourself, we want to allay your fears and again remind you that if C. diff hasn't killed you yet, it is very unlikely that it is ever going to kill you. Death from recurrent C. diff is rare. Most C. diff fatalities are first-time C. diff sufferers whose already compromised bodies were overwhelmed with the initial disease.

Whose fault is it?

Death is never fair, or particularly understandable, but when it happens to someone who is under the care of a doctor, it can be doubly vexing and challenge our cultural beliefs in doctors as heroes and miracle workers. C. diff-related deaths can be particularly shocking because they often occur unexpectedly. An elderly parent is admitted to the hospital for a broken hip, while there they develop pneumonia, and while being treated for pneumonia with antibiotics, they develop C.

diff. Suddenly, a relative with a simple broken bone is at death's door due to a microbe that you had not even heard of 24 hours ago. Anger is a natural reaction to this situation — anger and a need for answers. Why did this happen? Could it have been prevented? Who is responsible?

These are all understandable questions. They are also very tough questions to answer, particularly because without all the details of a specific case, anyone who addresses this topic is speaking in hypotheticals. We do know that there are a number of factors that can contribute to someone dying because of C. diff. Some of these factors are within the control of doctors, and the places where they work, and

You Can Help Beat the Beast! Interested in doing what you can to help beat the Beast? Consider giving money to an organization like the Peggy Lillis Memorial Foundation. The Foundation was started by Christian and Liam, sons of Peggy Lillis who succumbed to a C. diff infection in 2010. Christian and Liam honor their mother by raising money for the prevention of and education about C. diff. You can help them in this fight by finding them on the web at www.peggyfoundation.org and donating. C. diff is not a "sexy" disease. Bathroom diseases like it tend not attract a lot of attention or get talked about much in the media. Even if you don't have money to give, you can help educate others about C. diff by all becoming an advocate for the Peggy Lillis Foundation, and others like it, by telling your friends about it, forwarding their URL to folks you know, and asking for donations to the fund. A portion of the proceeds from the sale of this book go to support the foundation, so you've helped a little bit already!

some of them are not. We will address these issues in the form of the questions that are commonly asked after an adverse C. diff event, fatal or not.

Did the antibiotics I took give me (or my loved one) C. diff?

We wish we could give you a cut and dry answer here, but we cannot. Even though antibiotics are the most common culprit in initiating a C. diff infection, they are not the only one. In up to 80% of C. diff infections, antibiotics had been recently taken by the patient[8]. So it is possible, even likely, that the antibiotics were responsible for your C. diff, but it's also possible that they were just one instigator among many factors. In Chapter One we described a number of drugs and other factors that can contribute to C. diff. Exposure to any one of those drugs in the past three months could contribute to a C. diff infection. There are also the genetic issues involved. Patients are different, and the exact same set of factors that led to you getting C. diff might not cause any problem at all in another patient. Perhaps a more important question is, "should my loved one have been on antibiotics in the first place?" Keep in mind that most often the answer to this question is, "yes."

Could they have saved my loved one's life if they had diagnosed the C. diff earlier?

Another tough question to answer. It is possible that earlier identification of C. diff can lead to more positive outcomes. The problem in this case is the slowness of diagnostic tests (up to this point, at least; rapid DNA testing with the PCR test should eliminate this caveat soon) compared to the speed with which the disease can progress. In the past, diarrhea arising in the hospital, after antibiotics, might be assumed to be antibiotic-associated diarrhea, but not necessarily C. diff. Now, most hospitals will do a C. diff test immediately if a patient develops diarrhea after taking antibiotics. Even with more rapid diagnosis, the patients that are most susceptible to C. diff (the elderly, infirm, and immune-compromised) are also the ones most likely to develop paralytic ileus. Like other diarrheal diseases, C. diff can make a person very ill, very quickly, and sometimes C. diff simply moves too quickly for doctors and the drugs they prescribe to react.

When the Young and Healthy Die of C. diff.
Up to this point in the book we've done our best to allay the fears of death that many C. diff sufferers might have. We've taken this more optimistic route because we believe that more C. diff sufferers overestimate the risk of death from C. diff than underestimate it. We also know, from the research, that the majority of C. diff deaths occur in the elderly and infirm. Having said that, C. diff is a killer disease, and it does kill the young and healthy. Like its cousins MRSA and E. coli, C. diff can strike without warning and quickly overwhelm an otherwise healthy individual, killing them in a matter of days. The rise of newer, deadlier strains of C. diff has made this shocking occurrence more common. We hope this book allows you to better judge your personal risks from C. diff. Please don't obsess about dying of this disease, but please also take it very seriously. Even if you think of yourself as someone who couldn't possibly die of a diarrheal disease, listen to your gut. If it's telling you that something is dangerously not right, get yourself to a hospital immediately, communicate your concerns to someone who will listen and get yourself the treatment you need.

Could they have saved my loved one's life by preventing his initial infection with C. diff spores?

As we noted in Chapter One, many hospitals now quarantine patients with C. diff. The goal of this is to prevent non-infected patients from encountering C. diff spores. These practices do lead to reduction in the number of hospital-acquired C. diff infections, but they won't keep everyone from getting sick. Even with the best sanitation practices, some C. diff spores will be spread throughout the hospital. There are simply too many of them (billions upon billions), and they are too hardy to be completely killed with disinfectants. At this point, any hospital or long-term care facility comes with a risk, however small, of the presence of C. diff and possible infection if other factors are present.

Could alternative treatments have saved her life?

It is not unusual in terrifying circumstances for patients or their families to hunt for all possible treatments for an illness. Families of patients suffering from life-threatening C. diff infections may be frustrated that doctors aren't trying all of the alternative treatments described in this book. While we do believe that most of the alternative C. diff treatments described in this book (probiotics, sequestrants, etc.) can have a significant impact on patient recovery, it is important to remember that that impact is likely small compared to the benefit of the antibiotics all doctors will use to treat C. diff. The antibiotics (Flagyl, vancomycin, and others) are your real heavy hitters in the fight against C. diff. Secondly, it is important to remember that not all doctors are trained to implement the alternative treatments described here. The stool transplant, for example, can be an amazingly powerful tool in the hands of trained doctor, and a quite deadly one in the hands of an untrained one. A doctor who would gamble on a procedure that was unfamiliar to them would not be a responsible one.

Is it my fault for bringing my loved one here?

This is an easy one: no. No, it is not your fault for bringing your loved one to the hospital or long-term care facility where they got ill and ultimately perished. As we alluded to above, we would be shocked and amazed to find a health-care facility that was completely free of C. diff. Obviously, there was a good reason for taking your loved one to the health-care facility in the first place. If we were to avoid hospitals and nursing homes altogether because of the risk of infection, we would be doing ourselves and our families a disservice. As we have said multiple times throughout this book, there is no point in trading one illness for another, and we encourage you to make your health-care decisions based on a balanced measurement of the current and future risks.

Notes – Chapter Four

1. Redelings, M.D., Sorvillo, F., & Mascola, L. (2007). Increase in *Clostridium difficile*-related mortality rates, United States, 1999-2004. Emerging Infectious Diseases, 13(9): 1417.

2. Suda, V.A., (November 2010). Incidence and pedictors of acute kidney Injury in hospitalized *Clostridium difficile*-infected patients. A presentation to the American Society of Nephrology. Abstract TH-PO075.

3. Löffler, H.A., Pron, B., Mouy, R., Wulffraat, N.M., & Prieur, A-M. (2004). *Clostridium difficile*-associated reactive arthritis in two children. Joint Bone Spine, 71(1): 60.

4. Piche, T., Vanbiervliet, G., Pipau, F.G. (2007). Low risk of irritable bowel syndrome after *Clostridium difficile* infection. Canadian Journal of Gastroenterology, 21(11): 727.

5. Gerding, D.N, Johnson, S., Peterson, L.R., Mulligan, M.E., & Silva, Jr., J. (1995). *Clostridium difficile*-associated diarrhea and colitis. Infection Control and Hospital Epidemiology, 16: 459.

6. Piche et al, 2007.

7. Kenneally, C., Rosini, J.M., Skrupky, L.P., Doherty, J.A., Hollands, J.M., Martinez, E., McKenzie, W., Murphy, T., Smith, J.R., Micek, S.T., & Kollef, M.H. (2007). Analysis of 30-day mortality for *Clostridium difficile*-associated disease in the ICU setting. Chest, 132: 418.

8. Association for Professionals in Infection Control and Epidemiology. (2008). National Prevalence Study of *Clostridium difficile* in U.S. Healthcare Facilities. Washington, D.C.: APIC.

Chapter Five
The Future of C. difficile

As discussed in Chapter Five, the effects of C. diff can last long after the infection itself is gone. Besides the residual physical effects, many C. diff patients live with a lasting fear that their disease will return at any moment, with or without antibiotics. As we mentioned in Chapter Five, once enough time has passed since your last recurrence, it's highly unlikely that your C. diff will spontaneously return (assuming you are an otherwise healthy individual). It's likely that you will be able to take antibiotics again in the near or distant future without having another C. diff infection move in. Remember, a number of things have to happen for a C. diff infection to occur, and just because it happened once before doesn't mean it will happen again. However, we know that reassurance won't necessarily give you peace of mind, so what more can we offer you?

The Future of C. diff Prevention and Treatment

The good news is that research on C. diff has seen a real renaissance in the past ten years. In this chapter we'll talk about the exciting new developments that are likely to make C. diff a far rarer disease in the future, and one that is more easily treated.

Preventative Measures

Remember back in Chapter One when we talked about techniques for preventing C. diff? Well, these techniques aren't just for patients, hospitals are taking them to heart as well, and when they do so, C. diff infection rates fall. For example, in an April 16, 2009 article from the British newspaper *The Guardian*, it was reported that C. diff infection rates at British hospitals had dropped 38% from Fall 2007 to Fall 2008. What did British hospitals do to see this decrease? Two things: first, they educated their doctors and nurses on the importance of C. diff hygiene, and mandated hand washing instead of using alcohol-based disinfectants between seeing patients. Second, they educated doctors about the dangers of antibiotic oversubscription and got them to prescribe antibiotics only when they were truly needed. No more drugs for you if all you have is a cold or the flu! There were other factors involved here as well. Hospitals also did a better job quarantining infected patients and spent more money and time on disinfecting rooms and equipment that had been in contact with C. diff carriers. While it will be close to impossible to completely eradicate C. diff bacteria from hospitals, results like these show that fairly simple practices can have big returns in terms of lowering infection rates. Because results like

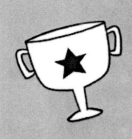

While on the job as a Fire Fighter/Medic, I was climbing over a metal gate in a barn when the hinges broke. The resulting drop left my knee with a six inch-wide laceration that had been exposed to animal manure. The doctors decided to use the most intense course of antibiotics at their disposal: Rocephin IV along with the maximum dosage of Cipro they could give. After about 2 weeks of this treatment, I began what was going to be a multi-year battle with C. diff.

Multiple attempts with Flagyl failed to cure me, so I sought out a gastroenterologist who conducted multiple colonoscopies. After a year of looking, he recommended that I have part of my colon removed. He took over ten inches of my colon, but my battle wasn't over; my C. diff remained. Over the next 15 months, using multiple courses of Vanco and chaser drugs, and an eventual Vanco taper, I finally seem to have beaten it. My story is an extreme example of particularly tough C. diff; it's not the norm, and I still beat it.

When you acquire C. diff you have a major infection in the largest, most complex system of organs in your body. The fact is that you will not beat it overnight, and your new post-C. diff normal may be totally different than pre-C. diff. The disease not only impacts us, but also our family and friends. Just a note though, the obsessive cleaning and bleaching is, (in my opinion) overkill...you are not a Typhoid Mary.

You can be a victim and let C. diff destroy and control your life or you can just be a person battling C. diff. The most difficult aspect of the battle for many is accepting the fact that you have finally gotten well. The other part is accepting the fact that not every stomach issue post C. diff is a relapse. We tend to forget that's a normal thing.

It's your responsibility to educate your doctors on the risks of overusing antibiotics, especially those that have been proven to cause C. diff. Do not hesitate to question a choice of drugs. Most doctors will work with you on the issue. When I had my neck rebuilt, I discussed the choice of antibiotics with him and his reply was, "well, then let's use Vanco."

"Fire" from the C. diff Support Site

these also save hospitals money, it's doubly likely they'll continue to invest in these practices.

New Antibiotics

Doctors and drug companies are constantly looking for new, more effective antibiotics. This search is largely driven by the bacteria themselves, who are constantly evolving resistance to existing drugs. As we've mentioned elsewhere in this book, the best antibiotics target only the bacteria that are hurting you at any given moment, and leave the rest alone. Doctors call these antibiotics "targeted," "narrow," or "tailored." It doesn't really matter what you want to call them, as long as you realize that to break the cycle of antibiotics and C. diff recurrence, it would be best to have an antibiotic that only killed the C. diff and let the rest of the gut flora recover normally.

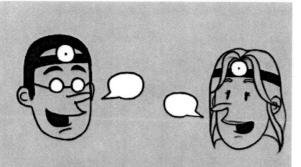

Off Label: When a doctor uses a drug "off label," they are using the drug for something it hasn't yet been approved for by regulating agencies, but they have good reasons and experience to suggest that the drug will be useful in that particular case.

There are a number of already on-the-market drugs (e.g. teicoplanin and rifaximin) that have not yet been approved by the FDA for use against C. diff, but in experimental studies have been found to be very effective against the bug. Many of these antibiotics are already being used off label by doctors to treat C. diff, and we can expect their approval and formal use soon. Keep in mind that gastroenterologists and infectious disease specialists are much more likely to be aware of these alternative antibiotics.

Because of the fickle nature of drug testing, new drugs in the development pipeline may sound promising one week and then be cancelled the next. So its important not to pin your hopes on the "next big thing." Having said that, there are some exciting new drugs in the pipeline that have been shown to have action against C. diff. One such narrowly-focused drug, fidaxomycin, was making C. diff headlines in early 2011 due to C. diff cure rates that were comparable to vancomycin, and recurrence rates that were significantly lower than vancomycin – as much as half the recurrence rates of vancomycin[1]! It's very difficult to predict when a drug that is still in testing, like fidaxomycin, is likely to make its way into doctors' offices, but it's worth asking your doctor about it if you aren't responding to current treatments as well as you'd like. To see an excellent summary of other new antibiotics (particularly some exciting new targeted antibiotics) in the development pipeline, see Monaghan, Boswell, & Mahida (2008)[2].

Germination: When doctors talk about bacterial germination, they're really talking about a process of change in the bacterial cell that changes it from a dormant spore to a creepy, crawly bacterium. It's easier just to think of it as hatching from something that can't hurt you, into something that can.

Spore Germinants

One of the more interesting treatments being considered for recurrent C. diff is the addition of chemicals called "spore germinants" to standard antibiotic treatments. Spore germinants force the germination of bacterial spores into active bacterial cells (also called vegetative cells) even when the bacteria normally wouldn't want to. The theory goes, if we can trigger all of the bacterial spores to germinate when antibiotics are being introduced into the system, all of the C. diff will be killed, and no spores will be around to lead to a recurrence of C. diff later[3]. A number of spore germinants are being developed and tested even as we write this book.

A C. diff vaccine

The holy grail of the fight against C. diff is a vaccine that keeps people from getting a C. diff infection even if they have been exposed to antibiotics and C. diff at the same time. Back in Chapter One we talked about those patients who seemed to have a stronger immune response to C. diff than others. Remember how those lucky people seemed to get over C. diff more quickly than others, or sometimes not get an active infection at all? Wouldn't it be great if we could make everyone like those people? That's what C. diff vaccine researchers are trying to do. While there are any number of ways to target a vaccine against C. diff, the most promising vaccines currently in development are "toxoid" vaccines, meaning they train your body to react to the C. diff toxin, not C. diff itself. This is the same way in which tetanus vaccines work, by the way, and as you'll recall, tetanus is caused by a close relative of C. diff: Clostridium tetani.

Clinicaltrials.gov: Should you find yourself in the very, very rare situation that current C. diff treatments, both mainstream and alternative, are not helping you, then you might consider looking for open clinical trials at clinicaltrials.gov. The website, maintained by the U.S. National Institutes of Health is a registry of all ongoing and proposed clinical trials in the U.S. Studies that are evaluating new drugs and treatments for efficacy will be listed here, along with information on who is eligible to enroll in the study and where they are enrolling members. At the time this book was being written, 40 different C. diff studies were listed on the site. Some of these were already complete, but many were open and enrolling patients.

Early trials with C. diff vaccines have been promising. Toxoid vaccines have been shown to induce a vigorous anti-toxin A antibody response in healthy volunteers injected with the vaccine[4]. And in a very small study, three patients with recurrent C. diff were cured and C. diff-free six months after being given a C. diff vaccine[5].

As of the writing of the first edition of this book in 2011, a C. diff vaccine is being developed by Sanofi-Pasteur, the vaccine production arm of Sanofi-Aventis, an internationally-based biotechnologies company. The C. diff vaccine had been fast-tracked by the Food and Drug Administration and was being studied in a Phase II clinical trial, meaning that it was being evaluated in a medium-sized group of patients (~650 in this case) for safety and efficacy at preventing first-time C. diff infections. Should the vaccine show promise in this trial, and acceptable side effects, then it would need to go into a Phase III trial in which it was tested on a much larger group of patients (between 1000 and 3000 typically). Assuming that all goes well with these trials, it's possible

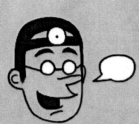

Clinical Trials Phases: The process of bringing a drug to market is a long and arduous one. New drugs must pass through several "phases" or hurdles that get progressively larger in scope and more complex in what is evaluated. Clinicaltrials.gov, a service of the U.S. National Institutes of Health offers this walkthrough of the various phases involved in testing a new drug:

"Most clinical trials are designated as phase I, II, III, or IV, based on the type of questions that study is seeking to answer:

In Phase I clinical trials, researchers test a new drug or treatment in a small group of people (20-80) for the first time to evaluate its safety, determine a safe dosage range, and identify side effects.

In Phase II clinical trials, the study drug or treatment is given to a larger group of people (100-300) to see if it is effective and to further evaluate its safety.

In Phase III clinical trials, the study drug or treatment is given to large groups of people (1,000-3,000) to confirm its effectiveness, monitor side effects, compare it to commonly used treatments, and collect information that will allow the drug or treatment to be used safely.

In Phase IV clinical trials, post marketing studies delineate additional information including the drug's risks, benefits, and optimal use.

These phases are defined by the Food and Drug Administration in the Code of Federal Regulations."

that a C. diff vaccine could be on the market as early as 2013 or 2014. We should add here, however, that there is no guarantee of a vaccine in this time frame. Testing new drugs and treatments for efficacy is a process fraught with false-starts and dead-ends.

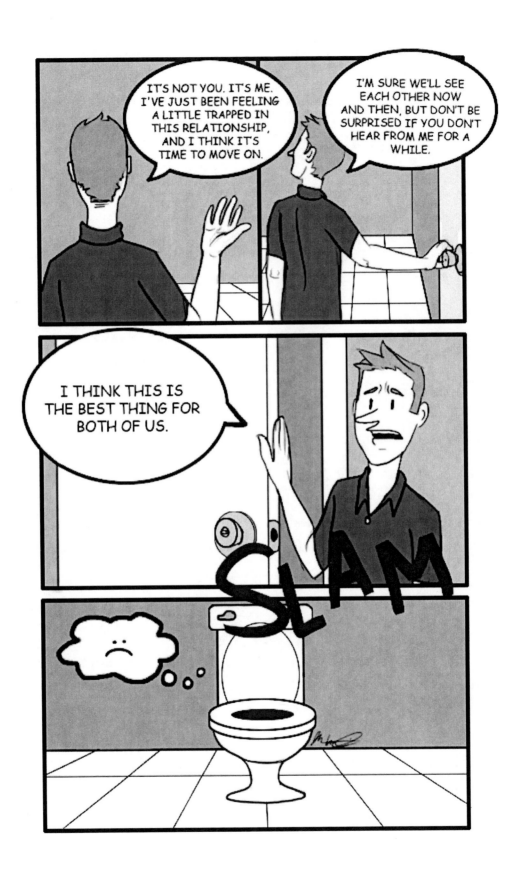

Even if a C. diff vaccine does make it to market, it may not work in everyone, and because it likely won't be given to all patients, it won't completely eradicate C. diff. However, we can imagine that just giving the vaccine to high-risk patients and those with highly recurrent C. diff could make a sizable dent in the prevalence of C. diff, and could potentially turn the disease from a real plague to a manageable nuisance that doctors and patients need not worry about too much. We are very hopeful for the success of this line of research.

Closing thoughts

We hope that this book has helped you to understand the nature of C. diff and the ways in which you and your doctor might address a C. diff infection.

We know that if you are currently suffering from recurrent C. diff, then you are likely in a very tough and lonely place. We want you to know that we understand the pain, suffering, and hopelessness that you must be feeling at times. We also want you to know that we honestly believe that you will get better. In our experience, everyone eventually gets over recurrent C. diff. For some it happens quicker, for some it happens slower, but in almost every case it happens.

So you've read the book, now what? Well, first, take a deep breath, get a hug from a loved one (or give one), and tell yourself that you are going to beat this disease. A positive attitude (with some humor mixed in, if you can manage it) is key to a more tolerable recovery. Second, think about having a conversation with your doctor about your various treatment options. If you're not yet on a tapered pulse, talk to your doctor about when you might start one. If you've been on a tapered pulse, and it didn't work, talk to your doctor about some of the other options mentioned in Chapter 3.

Lastly, and perhaps most importantly, connect to the community of C. diff sufferers online. The biggest community that we know of is at www.cdiffsupport.com. Log on, share your story, and learn what others are doing to treat their disease. The emotional support you'll get there, as well as the information and guidance, is priceless. Someday, we promise you, you're going to be logging on to the forums to share your story of how you beat the Beast.

Notes – Chapter Five

1.   Louie, T.J., Miller, M.A., Mullane, K.M., Weiss, K., Lentnek, A., Golan, Y., Gorbach, S., Sears, P., & Shue, Y-K. (2011). Fidaxomicin versus vancomycin for *Clostridium difficile* infection. The New England Journal of Medicine, 364: 422.

2.   Monaghan, T., Boswell, T., & Mahida, Y. (2008). Recent advances in *Clostridium difficile*-associated disease. Gut, 57: 850.

3.   Sorg, J.A. & Sonenshein, A.L. (2008). Bile salts and glycine as co-germinants of *Clostridium difficile*. Journal of Bacteriology, 190(7): 2505.

4.   Kotloff, K.L., Wasserman, S.S., Losonsky, G.A., Tohomas, W.J., Nichols, R., Edelman, R., Bridwell, M., & Monath, T.P. (2001). Safety and immunogenicity of increasing doses of a *Clostridium difficile* toxoid vaccine administered to healthy adults. Infection and Immunity, 69: 988 and Aboudola, S., Kotloff, K.L., Kyne, L., Warny, M., Kelly, E.C., Sougioultzis, S., Giannasca, P.J., Monath, T.P., Kelly, C.P. (2003). *Clostridium difficile* vaccine and serum immunoglobulin G antibody response to toxin A. Infection and Immunity, 71: 1608.

5.   Sougioultzis, S., Kyne, L., Drudy, D., Keates, S., Maroo, S., Pothoulakis, C., Giannasca, P.J., Lee, C.K., Warny, M., Monath, T.P., & Kelly, C.P. (2005). *Clostridium difficile* toxoid vaccine in recurrent C. *difficile*-associated diarrhea. Gastroenterology,128: 764.

Appendix A: The Big Takeaways

1. C. diff most often occurs after exposure to antibiotics in the hospital or another disturbance to the gut's natural bacterial flora.

2. New strains of C. diff are emerging that are more potent, more deadly, and more resistant than the strains we have seen up to this point. Although still less common than hospital-acquired C. diff, it is becoming more and more common to become infected with C. diff outside of the hospital, and without having taken antibiotics.

3. C. diff kills about 1%-2% of those it infects.

4. Hand washing, isolation of infected patients and sterilization of shared equipment and spaces look to be the best ways to prevent the spread of C. diff in hospitals and long-term care facilities.

5. The majority of C. diff patients will be cured with one or two doses of an antibiotic.

6. A minority (15-30%) will suffer from repeated recurrences of the infection.

7. Taking probiotics whenever you take antibiotics may help prevent an initial infection of C. diff, and may help prevent recurrences of C. diff.

8. A majority of these recurrent C. diff sufferers will be cured with more antibiotics, typically delivered in a tapered-pulsed dose.

9. Complementary treatments (antibiotic chasers, immune boosters, stool transplants) may help recurrent C. diff sufferers recover more quickly without further recurrences.

10. The future of C. diff treatment looks bright. New drugs, different modes of treatment, and a vaccine against C. diff look quite possible in the near future.

11. If you are in the middle of a C. diff infection, or suffering from multiple recurrences, you will get over it eventually.

12. We mean it. You will get over it eventually.

13. C. diff hates it when you laugh at it. We promise. Laugh at it as much as you can.

CPSIA information can be obtained at www.ICGtesting.com
Printed in the USA
BVOW050825011211

277369BV00002B/2/P